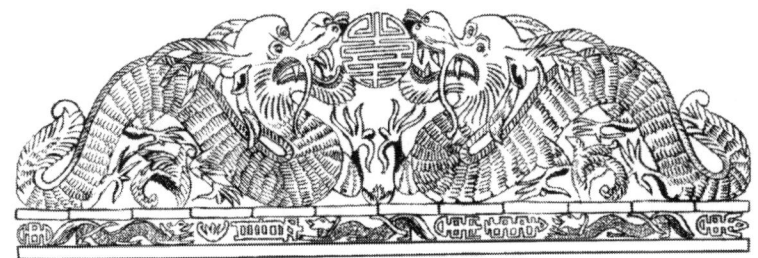

Tai Chi
Students Confessions continued

Up close
And
Personal

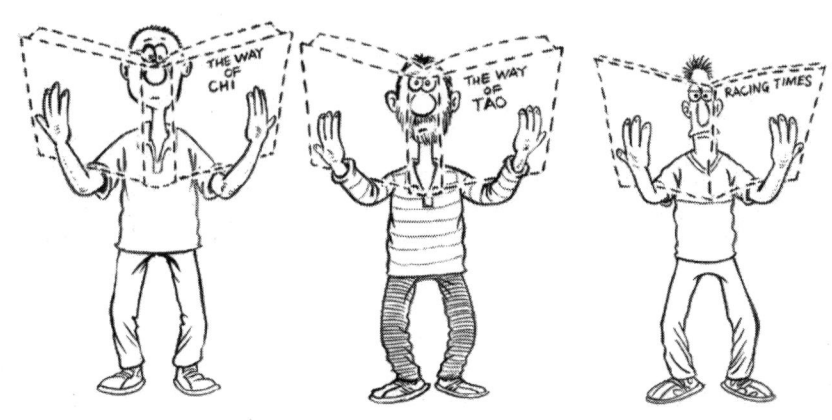

Copyright ©2015 Kai Ming Association for Tai Chi Chuan

All rights reserved. This work may not be copied in any manner whatsoever without the permission of the publisher, except for short extracts for the purpose of review.

We would like to dedicate this book to all teachers and students past, present and yet to be, for giving us the motivation to produce this book and continue the journey.
Mark & Jenny Peters

Cartoons and cover by Hunt Emerson: Largecow.com

ISBN-13:
978-1519379009

ISBN-10:
1519379005

Introduction

It has been seven years since we published our first book **'Views from the back of the** class' and so we thought that maybe it was time to share some further views and experiences from the students and instructors that hopefully will again inspire new and experienced Tai Chi players alike.

The diversity of the articles within this second book, and the people who wrote them, is vast; many of the chapters have been submitted by students and teachers who contributed to the first book and are still with us.

We hope it will make for another interesting read.

There is a plethora of instructional form books, and even more deeply interesting theory and practice of Tai Chi literature; they have a recognized place in a practitioners reading.

However sometimes reading people's personal experiences and feelings can trigger you to delve deeper into a certain area of Tai Chi; a trigger to exploring your own thoughts and experiences.
With this in mind we included an Epilogue that contains a selection of writings that although not obviously linked to Tai Chi we thought you may enjoy, and where submitted to us for our monthly club newsletter by students and instructors.

We are hoping, we have, as before, structured the chapters to ensure this tai chi book is a 'dip in' easy read, and often light-hearted view of tai chi life.

Jenny Peters

Table of Contents

Introduction — 4

Part 1 - Push-hands: up close and personal — 13

Push Hands Without Force? Something to Ponder. — 14
Mark Peters

A Pianist's Touch — 17
Jenny Peters

Rooting and Its Dynamics. — 18
Mark Peters

Anger Within Push Hands — 21
Mark Peters

The Push Hands Connection — 24
Jenny Peters

Master Li Yaxuan's Explanatory Notes on Push Hands — 26
translated by Scott Meredith

My Students Don't Want To Do Push Hands — 30
Mark Peters

A point to Reflect on — 33
Mark Peters

Hands— The Fine Tools Of Internal Arts — 35
Jenny Peters

Energy Forward Corresponding Movement Backward — 36
Mark Peters

Chinese Character Yan (Ren) — 37
Mark Peters

Part 2 - Meditation & Mindfulness — 38

A Meditation For You To Try — 39
Jenny Peters

On Teaching 41
Kahlil Gibran

The Miracle of Mindfulness 42
Mark Peters

An Introduction to Meditation 44
Mark Walker

Stillness 48
Jenny Peters

Meditation part 2 50
Mark Walker

Inner Peace: This is so true 52
Anonymous

Chinese Proverbs - The Chinese Puzzle Unravelled 53
Jenny Peters

Movement and stillness conspired one day 55
Jenny Peters

How To Get The Best From Your Brain 57

Oh... to sit quietly 58
Mark Peters

Breathing And The Mind 59
William Cc Chen

Believe Nothing 61
Anonymous

Part 3 – Health 62

Values. 63
Anonymous

How To Be Happy In 18 Easy Steps 64
Dalai Lama

Tai Chi Helps You Sleep Better. 66
Anonymous

Preparing To Practice Qigong.   67
Jenny Peters

Talking Alignment. A Word From The Converted   69
Jenny Peters

How Tai Chi exercises benefit the knee joint   72
Mark Peters

Qigong - Get Started.   74
Jenny Peters

Before Tai Chi   77
Ron Davies

Keeping The (Your) Balance   83
Jenny Peters

The Quiet Corner   85

Banish those aches and pains   86

Tai-Chi "Soaking It In" !   87
Jenny Peters

Strange But True - Joint Points   89

Balance Comes From Many Skills.   90
Mark Peters

3 Pressure Points to Heal Yourself   93
Mao Shing Ni

The Big B!—— And How To Avoid It.   95
Jenny Peters

Have you got the spine for it?   99
Mark Peters

Learn To Walk Before You Run   101
Mark Peters

A Black Bag Job -- Sue's Story   104
Sue Priece

Part 4 – Tai Chi Journeys	108
Teaching, Stress and Chinese Martial Arts *David Jones*	109
PASSION - Strong emotion, strong enthusiasm. *Jenny Peters*	111
Tai Chi Chainsaw *Nigel Holt*	113
My Tai Chi Journey *Leigh Mathers*	115
Neglecting the near in search of the far - Part 1 *Jenny Peters*	118
An instructor's view… Part 2 *Mark Peters*	121
I'm in Ron's Group *Mark Peters*	123
A Students Journey *Mick Tucker*	126
A View From The Front Of The Class *Neil Rankine*	127
Ben Lee's Story *Ben Lee*	131
Learning Tai Chi In Unexpected Circumstances *Josie Upson*	134
Martial Art Moses? *Jenny Peters*	137
The Ego-climber *Mark Peters*	141
The Tai Chi Instructor (Smooth Operator) *Jacqui d'Auban*	143
My Journey From The Back Of The Class To The Front *Lynne Jenkins*	144

Ward Off Right With A Zimmer Frame	146
Jayne Wilson	
Rainbows End	148
Jenny Peters	
Part 5 – Form & Function	152
KAI MING (Open Minded)	153
Jenny Peters	
Alice In Wonderland And Tai Chi!	155
Jenny Peters	
The Bubbling Well.	158
Mark Peters	
On Teachers And Training	160
Jenny Peters	
Important Points	161
Mark Peters	
Training tips	162
Mark Peters	
Subtle skills of tai chi	163
Mark Peters	
Balance And Coordination	165
Mark Peters	
The Form	167
mark Carter	
Points on Using The Principles of Tai Chi.	169
Jenny Peters	
Inside Out Martial Arts	172
Ben Ford	
Are There Circles And Squares In Tai Chi?	174
Anonymous	
A Beginners Guide To Class Confusion	176
Ian Anderson	

There Is No Transition *Alan Sanson*	180
Tai Chi And The Element Of Relaxation. *Jenny Peters*	181
Yang Style Tai Chi Chuan Twenty-Character Motto *Yang Zhenduo*	183
The Riddle of the Tai Chi Classics *Don Morgan*	185
The importance of Dong-Dang (swing-return) *Mark Peters*	186
The Waist And its Importance in Tai Chi Practice. *Jenny Peters*	187
The Inner Game *Mark Peters*	189
Q&A From Huang Sheng-Shyan (Huang Xingxian)	191
The Importance Of The Five Loosening Exercises *Willie Lim*	193
Q&A From Huang Shengshyan (Huang Xingxian)	195
Q&A From Huang Sheng-Shyan (Huang Xingxian)	197
Q&A From Huang Sheng-Shyan (Huang Xingxian)	200
Low Punch (the lowdown) *Jenny Peters*	202
Getting it right *Mark Peters*	205
Q&A On Tao Of Tai Chi Chuan. By Master Huang Sheng Shyan	206
The Empowering Principles of Tai Chi *Jenny Peters*	207
Dance to the Beat of Tai Chi *Hunt Emerson*	210

Rooting, Chi And The Mind. *Mark Peters*	212
Stability *Jenny Peters*	214
Am I in a Tai Chi Trance? *Mark Peters*	216
Some Things Don't Change Or Do They? *Jenny Peters*	219
Training Method For Tai Chi Chuan *Yang Ban Hou*	221
Passing On The Art *Jenny Peters*	223
Q&A On Tao Of Tai Chi Chuan. By Master Huang Sheng Shyan	225
For what Purpose? *Jenny Peters*	227
Part 6 – Martial Application	228
The Art Of Not Fighting? *Jenny Peters*	229
Q&A From Huang Sheng-Shyan (Huang Xingxian)	233
Tai Chi Chuan—Boxing for the Gentle *Senyung Chow*	236
Training The Mind's Eye *Jenny Peters*	245
Elements Of Combatitive Tai Chi Chuan *Anonymous*	246
Stillness In The Martial Arts *Ted Mancuso*	248
Tai Chi The Non-Discriminative Art *Jenny Peters*	250

Putting The "Chuan" Back In Tai Chi Chuan *Jenny Peters*	255
The Dying Art of "Stillness" *Jenny Peters*	260
Part 7 – Epilogue – Beyond Tai Chi	262
Thought For The Day... *Jenny Peters*	263
A story for Christmas.. *Colonel John Mansur*	264
A Pause For Thought *Jenny Peters*	266
Chi, the Universe and Nan's Voodoo Wart Cure *Rob Charteris*	267
How To Please A Monkey! *Mark Peters*	270
Pearls Of Wisdom Advice From My Mother ! *Jenny Peters*	272
The History Of Boading Balls *Jenny Peters*	273

Part 1 - Push-hands: up close and personal

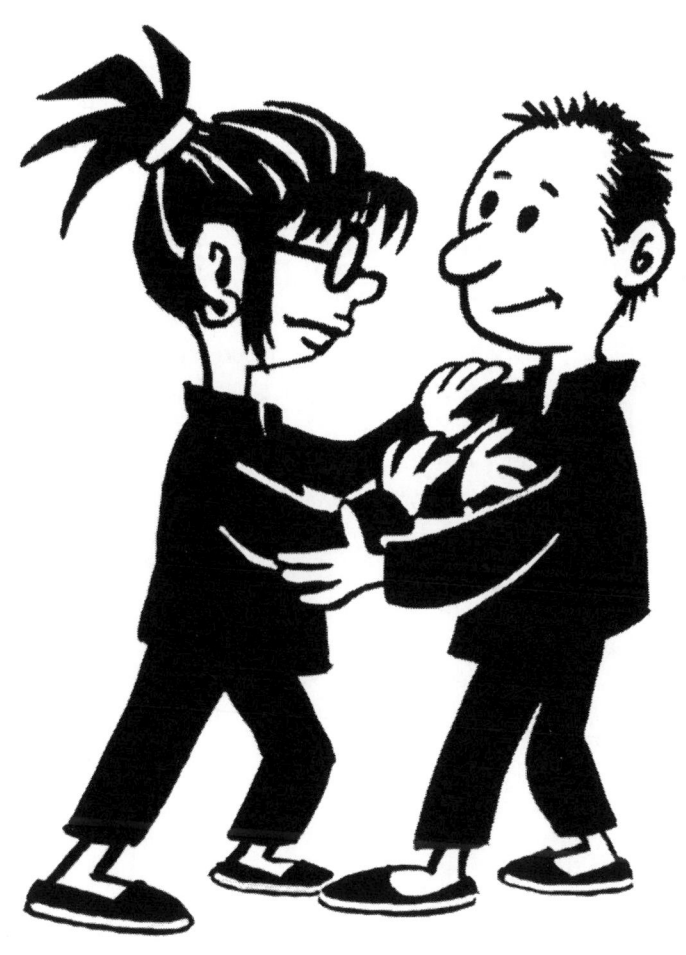

Push Hands Without Force? Something to Ponder.

Theories abound regarding the intricacies of Push Hands, and I believe there is no easy answer to how to disengage the muscles. After all since time began they have been receiving messages from the brain to function in one way.
Tai Chi asks them to sometimes do the opposite, i.e. don't tighten up to give more force, relax, and get a better result.
Line up the joints, free up the hips and waist, feel grounded through the feet, and last but not least focus the mind on what you hope to achieve - effortless power.
William C. C. Chen in his 1999 article "The Mechanics of Three Nails" writes "Not until in the middle 80's that I began to realize that the thigh itself has no ability to make any moves or turns without the help of the foot which is rooted firmly on the ground. Therefore, the rooted foot, and specifically the "three active nails" are in control and energized…"
Turning, therefore, starts from the feet. As the feet "turn", they cause the hips to turn. .

This is the point where many students fail, because they do not connect and move as a unit. The body turns but the arms do not follow.
Your arms must stay in front of your body and move with it at all times. The space under the armpits must not close and your arms must not collapse against your sides.
Another aspect of turning that is very important is the hip joint (KUA) must be sunk and the front knee bent.
If this is not done the front knee and kua almost straighten out, in turn the entire side of the body from the ankle to the shoulder becomes a straight line.
Accordingly the hip will rise along the centre of gravity, and the root will disappear causing instability and leaving you an easy prey for your opponents push.

As we all know a good root is essential, whether in Tai Chi or everyday life.

I have heard someone say to understand how to sink and root, imagine holding a plastic bag that is two-thirds filled with water, the bottom is heavy and pulls downward, while the further up the bag that you go the lighter and lighter it gets.
Beginners often rush to push their opponent. Push hands calls for patience, the right moment, the opportunity and finding a weakness Expansion is the key to enabling you to make your partner unbalance themselves.
Joseph Eber a teacher from New Jersey explains what is known as "THE PYTHON EFFECT" which is the basis of the above.
The python squeezes its prey so that the prey cannot expand its lungs to breathe. With every exhale, the snake tightens its coils, preventing the prey from taking in a breath, until all oxygen in its lungs is exhausted.
Like the snake, when you sense a weakness, expand into it and stay there. Your opponent will attempt to move in another direction, usually back-wards to escape your expansion.
When they do that, they will create another weakness somewhere else.
Expand into it as well without letting up.

Pretty soon your opponent will run out of places to move. They will become immobilized as you keep expanding into them until they lose their footing.
To put it simply, the more you expand, the less your opponent can expand, and if they cannot expand and keep their joints open, including the lower back, then they will lose power along with their balance.

When pushed instinct often makes us do the opposite to expanding, instead we shrink our posture. We stiffen up and react by pulling our arms into our body.
Notice what happens when you are moved off balance or seconds before you are moved. Many of you will realise you where pulling the other players arm into you therefore helping them to move your root and in turn take your balance.

Remember at all times RELAX AND EXPAND. (Peng - ward off)
After all we should be doing this every time we do the form.

Cheng Man Ching said "everything comes from the form"

So whether you are practising the straight sword, broad sword, fan, stick, staff or push hands remember these wise words.

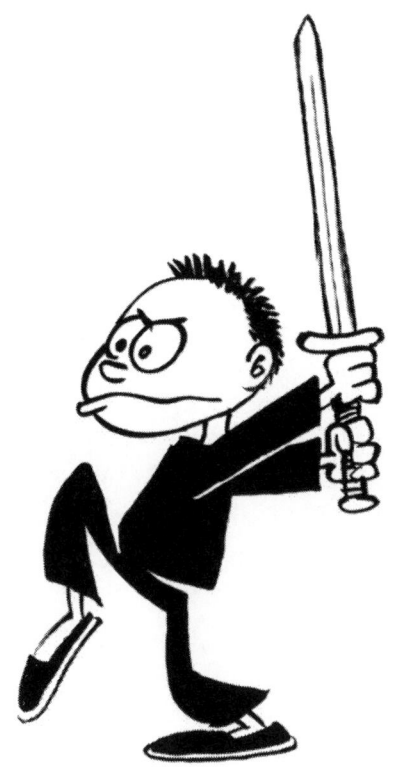

A Pianist's Touch

(thoughts on powers of relaxation)
Claudio Arrau the great pianist (1903-1991), a native of Chile, was a child prodigy who had his debut at the age of five. Known as a remarkably thorough and expressive musician, he kept to a rigorous practice and touring schedule his whole life. Arrau spent years carefully analyzing the movements involved in piano-playing. He advocated keeping relaxed and letting the weight of the body and gravity do most of the work. Arrau was able to practice for up to fourteen hours a day without fatigue, in part due to his ability to keep relaxed.

In an interview late in life Arrau said,

"If you keep your body relaxed, the body is in contact with the depths of your soul. If you are stiff in any joint, you impede the current, the emotion, the physical current - what the music itself dictates to you - if you are not relaxed, you won't be able to let it go through into the keyboard".

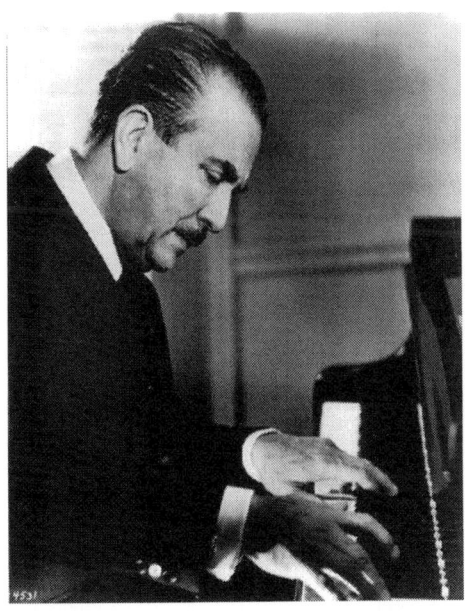

Rooting and Its Dynamics.

Rooting is one of the greatest points of confusion in the Tai Chi player's training. It seems extremely hard to get any sort of concrete instruction in this matter, beyond mystical visualization.
Compounding this is the tendency to define skills by their success in certain limited contexts; in this case tui-shou (push hands)
However subtle receiving energy can only be used if the opponent is motivated by the threat of ordinary attack.
It is normally of little significance because normal attacks come from people using their body in a relatively normal way.
As Cheng Man Ching remarked: "Even the highest technique cannot discharge a statue!"
William Chen told how Cheng had a rather special class for a few of his best students, to acquaint them with some higher levels of fa-jin. Everything went fine for the first few weeks, but then a peculiar thing happened. Suddenly it seemed that Cheng could no longer make his discharges work. He seemed to lose his power.
The professor gathered them together for a talk.
He explained to them that in the beginning, they had been afraid of him, uncertain as to what was going to happen, and had therefore manifested plenty of energy in resisting his attacks.
(I wonder if this "energy" was in fact fear making them tense and therefore much easier to uproot)
Now, he explained, they all had gotten to know him and realized that they were in no real danger. The greatest master of receiving energy can do nothing when there is no energy to receive.
They had, he explained further, a choice. Either they could start exhibiting the kind of reactions and energy appropriate to a fearful situation, or he would have to start actually hurting them in order to produce such sincerity.
In the examples above this annoying stagnancy is, on the one hand, a part of an unhealthy psychological condition, and on the other, a simple accident of misunderstanding.
It is common to see players "relax" their upper bodies into a kind of undifferentiated stagnancy, and then use their legs to launch this like a projectile at their opponent.

This kind of stagnancy gives them, when not attacking, a kind of root, but comparable with the correct one in the way that a large heavy object, like a safe, compares with a tree. The safe is "rooted" solely by virtue of its weight and its frictional pressure on the floor. The tree may be comparatively light in weight, but its attachment to the ground makes it difficult to move.

It is common to characterize some players using techniques with having a "good root".

In fact, the highest technique is enjoyed by one who can skilfully neutralize both pressure and rotational forces in the feet and make pressure appear on the ground only after all neutralization has been exhausted.

Force from the opponent may come not only in a linear form, but also have twisting, rotational components.

The movement of the player receiving such force must be such that all force is neutralized to the degree that no evidence of it may be found in the connection between the feet and the floor.

One of the most profound truths of Tai Chi Chuan is that the apparent goal of Tai Chi, that is, the reflection or emanation of great force in the direction of the opponent, is actually the opposite of the goal that one must actually pursue, which is the neutralization or absorption of force.

It is only by the exhaustion of this effort that one arrives at the proper condition for discharge.

This is more in keeping with the old concept of "walking on snow without leaving tracks!"

Discharge is more an accident of good technique than the result of deliberate attempts to do so.

To understand the connection between root and winding forces, we need to think back to its earliest form, it was then referred to as "breaking the root" not uprooting.

Also the earliest form of discharge was known as long discharge.

The opponent would be thrown down and backwards along the floor, rather than "up in the air and away"

This was achieved by the use of winding energy in a forceful way.

If you pull a plant from the earth, to get better leverage you probably pull and twist at the same time. This makes it much easier than a straight pull.

Winding energy such as this deployed on an opponent peels his feet from the floor (breaking the root) before he is thrown, and looks quite impressive.

Although this technique may "do the job" the price paid for continual use of this method may be the loss of some control over the situation, where the practitioner may choose to show his mastery by simple "rooting in," and becoming immovable, or even "discharging" one's opponent.

Therefore it is really important that rootedness not become defined simplistically as heaviness or immovability.

Rootedness is only achieved correctly when it is coordinated with other skills which are of equal importance.

If you rely on "set tactics" they will depend entirely on maintenance of a set of specific rules which will not translate well to real fighting.

Tai Chi needs "spirit" not techniques, it needs "feeling and sensing" not ego and strength.

If you do not develop these skills then your tai chi will come to a dead end and stagnate.

Skill brings a great aliveness to the feet and the sensation that, no matter how fast one moves, even when just walking, there is control of balance, which transfers to the whole body as each foot makes contact with the floor.

You will not acquire your root by imitation of the state of consciousness of someone who has found theirs.

It will not magically appear this way.

In fact, the consciousness of the master of these skills is characterized by the fact that he has forgotten them!

Rootedness is not the skill.

Proper leg movement and body balance is the skill, and rootedness, the describable result

Anger With in Push Hands

"Did you ever feel your temper flare while doing push hands with a difficult partner? Whenever it happens to me, it catches me by surprise because the taijiquan (Tai Chi Chuan) philosophy of gentleness and yielding is contrary to the sudden violence and 'stuckness' of anger" - JAN NYE teacher of Tai Chi Chuan in Minneapolis.

Anger is the word we've chosen to use to describe the emotion/sensation each of us has experienced in push-hands when the experience is not what was expected or our planned outcome isn't happening. You may call it frustration, not wanting to lose (investing in loss), fear or many other things... automatic reflex even.... Above all, it is a fight-or-flight response that is no longer useful. One instructor made a chance remark recently for which I am very grateful, as it made me consider how students may view push hands in all classes; they said **"I'm not interested in push-hands, I'm not interested in the martial aspects of tai chi, nor are my students"**. This idea can be seen as a natural one but is actually born out of a lack of understanding of the true nature of physical and mental balance; with anger and fear at their core. Tai Chi is being extensively studied for patient rehabilitation and one key area of study is falls prevention. It has been proven that fear of falling increases the risk of falling significantly. Push-hands is a perfect tool to improve balance and stability through proprioception and kinaesthesia. We have had students with peripheral neuropathy come to tai chi to reduce falls; push-hands has been a great tool as it is a method of training balance awareness feedback which can be used to take another person's balance or help them find it. Anger, frustration and fear are close bed-fellows. Here is a quote from one of my favourite books, Dune (1965)

"I must not fear. Fear is the mind-killer. Fear is the little-death that brings total obliteration. I will face my fear. I will permit it to pass over me and through me. And when it has gone past I will turn the inner eye to see its path. Where the fear has gone there will be nothing. Only I will remain."

Push-hands is the perfect vehicle to explore and deal with Anger in a safe and controlled/structured environment. Anyone who has practiced push-hands a number of times would have experienced this and it can be seen as a natural occurrence of two people facing each other and trying to push each other over, even without intended force. Stiffening, resisting, grabbing when your balance is lost, using more force than should be necessary etc are all signs of anger and are a chance to learn, experience and understand this emotion. Push-hands is a physical and psychological negotiation that requires keenly developed listening skills; these listening skills enable the exponent to accept, neutralise and lead the interaction seemingly effortlessly. Is this not the skills of a good negotiator? Anger throws a wall up and creates opposition not negotiation. Anger does not create space for response. In the five elements of Chinese Medicine, the emotion opposite anger is sympathy (consideration). It may be a long road from anger to sympathy but in listening to each other, as the tai chi principles ask us to do, aren't we being sympathetic? Our anger can actually dissolve as we move towards sympathy. Applying the idea of **'do not insist, do not resist'** asks that we stay with what is happening, be mindful and listen.

A great tool for dealing with anger in push-hands is a change of perspective where the opponent is no longer seen as an opponent but as a teacher; the more force they apply the more we can learn to neutralise or to 'invest in loss'. Please remember force cannot be applied if there is nothing to apply force to, so you must be creating a point of resistance for them to push against…..

Push-hands helps you find your feet. I often say "The only thing you need to do in tai chi is to not fall over!" To expand on this I mean not fall over your body but fall into it, into your feet, so you enable natural compression and balance. A push should only push you into your feet enabling you to relax into balance. Anger activates the wrong muscle groups and creates lines of resistance both mentally and physically.

By helping us find our feet in push-hands we find our feet in life; there is a great story of Yang Cheng-Fu walking down a road and talking with friends when a stranger ran past and bumped into him; the stranger rebounded off and flew a great distance whilst Yang Cheng-Fu didn't even break his conversation – he had found his feet. When we consider how often we mentally or physically bump into others in our life, creating potential anger opportunities or opportunities to learn patience; my one teacher (Koh Ah Tee) often refers to tai chi as patience boxing. Practice 'patience under pressure' and listen as new opportunities present themselves. There is no shortcut to this learning only practice. There is a long route though…. Hold on to your anger and see where that takes you, put it down and see where it leads, the choice is always yours…

The Push Hands Connection

George Xu said in an article I read that the development of high level martial skills in Tai Chi Chuan involves cultivating the ability to connect one's own intention with the intention of the opponent, according to Wang Hao Da, disciple of the late and great Ma Yueh-Liang.

Wang has exceptional push hands skills from his training with Ma and his own research

He believes if you can match your own intention, or yi, with that of your opponent you follow this through by harmonizing with them in such a way that the two become one so that you can direct the opponent's movement.

You conceal your own intention and energy so that they cannot control you.

Wang adds this skill is acquired by practicing the form, creating a strong, lively, needle-like centre of equilibrium (zhong ding) that the opponent can't find.

This point is re-enforced continually within Kai-ming as it is one of Mark's founding principles as a young! Trainee.

Grand Master Ma's method is based on his key points of: Don't use strength; use quality, but not jin; use the invisible, not the visible, and use the internal, not the external.

This will in turn create the deep centre of equilibrium that Ma could rely on for strength instead of external force.

This gave him pliability and looseness to repulse forceful attacks.

Qiao means a well- trained body.

From letting others in training touch and push you, you can become skilful in 'knowing' them.

You will find their centres; feel their power and the size of it.

However remember the other "player" may be seeking the same within you.

A lot will depend on which one of you is prepared to invest in loss or "eat bitter" and therefore let go of ego.

By yielding and dissolving your internal strength (Jin) you can absorb others' power and become like a compressed spring, ready to release back at them.

Qiu means to probe your own root. It needs to be made strong for you to use folding power and issuing power correctly and to your best advantage.

Your root has to be strong (natural and effortless) and your hips have to be loose, so that you can "appear and disappear" at will, and to your opponents confusion!

To relax and sink in Ma's opinion was not enough to have a good root.

To "nail it" you need to screw down into the earth using your yi and qi

A lot of people have internal energy, but they cannot connect it to the external movement and deliver it.

The inside and outside remain separate.

Working on your form you can develop the answer to this problem of what is effectively 'your transmission'.

Internal strength should always be present in the form. You must move through the form with your body whilst your inside is 'alive'.

Wang recalls Ma (who he studded with for 21 years) was always calm, mentally open and strong. He never rushed, was peaceful, never anxious.

He took the 'middle way'. Never eating too much, he was steady happy and pleasant whenever he met someone. All his practice was internal, pure internal

For Ma, the internal was always the major.

The internal was always activated first, before the external body.

This is the Chinese martial art at its highest level.

It is said that when Ma lightly touched you, you started to 'float'.

It was because the quality of his sinking was so great that it neutralized your root.

He told Wang "there are a thousand kinds of change and a million kinds of neutralization.

Changing, he said, is easy since it is external and may mean just changing position. But to disappear inside, there are a million different ways. Hua-jin neutralization is a much higher level of skill than changing."

Ma's reputation will live on as one of the real and humble Master's and his practice and dedication to the form, (even continuing into old age) was the secret to this great man.

Maybe it can be yours?

Master Li Yaxuan's Explanatory Notes on Push Hands

translation by Scott Meredith.

Master Li Yaxuan was the most accomplished senior student of Grandmaster Yang Cheng fu, and he was a senior classmate of Professor Zheng Manqing (Cheng Man Ching).

From the moment of contact with my partner's hands, I am using the lively emptiness and lightness of my own hands to follow his every move. As I follow, before he knows it my presence has infiltrated his body. From this point onward, the slightest movement of my spirit energy and activation of my dan-tian's qi store will immediately send him reeling as though he's touched a live electric wire. What we call emptiness contains everything, and what we call liveliness feels all, so that whenever the right opportunity comes to your hands your internal energy's automatic reaction instantly sends him sprawling out. Therefore, in pushing hands you need not seek out a particular time or chance to push him, no need to force anything. When the chance has perfectly developed on its own, you'll feel that jump straight into your hands. Very rarely you will not feel that chance come to you right away, and this just means that no fault is yet apparent in your partner's energy. In this case, there's no need for you to try to force an opening or forcefully oppose him, you should simply maintain your alert hands. If after a long period you cannot detect any flaw in him, it may be that his level is higher than yours. Then you should humbly seek instruction from him, to further your own knowledge. Struggling to force a victory won't do anything to develop your skill.

Once, somebody asked Grandmaster Yang Cheng-fu the following: "We never see you putting on any big show of power, so how is it that you can blast people such a distance with such sharp focus?" Grandmaster Yang replied: "It's because I am issuing relaxed energy." Somebody else asked Grandmaster Yang Shao-hou the following: "You seem so relaxed when you issue energy, how can that possibly be so powerful?" Grandmaster Yang replied: "It's precisely because I'm relaxed that my energy is so effective." The replies of these two teachers establish very clearly that relaxation is the unalterable foundation of Taijiquan both for push hands and combative applications.

Ward-off, rollback, press, push; plucking, splitting, elbowing, shouldering; advancing, retreating, looking right, looking left; and centring - these are the 13 basic motions of Taijiquan, and they must be conscientiously applied. As for adhering, following, and the principles of no gaps and no resistance - these are even more important to research thoroughly. You must relentlessly pursue these ideas or you'll never understand real taijiquan and you'll just end up wasting your time.

The idea of adhering doesn't only refer to the physical touching of hands. Even before your hands make contact, cover the opponent or partner entirely with your spirit and modulate your breath in accordance with his motions of extending and withdrawing - this is the deeper meaning of adherence. As you follow and track his motions, your hands have subtly and quietly come to the point of controlling his body. Then you'll be able to manipulate his every move to your own advantage.

The three principles of adherence:
1. As soon as the slightest physical contact is made, you must listen to his expansions and
contractions and follow them - this is called tactile adherence.
2. Before physical contact is made, you must observe and judge the distance between you and position yourself accordingly - this is called visual adherence.
3. You must learn to listen for the features of his voice that help you to judge distance and to
position yourself accordingly - this is called aural adherence.

All of the above are dependent on the cultivation of a sensitive and lively spirit, which is the
most fundamental concern of Taijiquan training. All of Taijiquan push hands is based on ward-off, rollback, press, and push, which embody the ideas of no gaps and no resistance, so that every time you touch with light sensitivity and the softness of cotton. If you don't properly distinguish ward-off, rollback, press, and push or if your touch is strong and hard, then that's external boxing.

You should approach push hands with a light and alert spirit. Though you may have some
combative skills don't use them against him. Though you may have some techniques, don't use those either. You must use your spirit to neutralize and counter. to make him feel he's chasing the wind and grasping at shadows, as though he has nowhere solid to stand, as though there's nowhere to run, nowhere to hide, let him defeat himself with his own actions, then he'll be easily overcome. If you try to use techniques to block or counter his motions and attacks, he'll be able to forestall your application of whole-body energy and all your efforts will be clumsy and futile. Pay attention to this.

You must not contaminate your practice by continuing at the same time with external or physical methods of training and attempt to apply those to your push hands practice. This is absolutely pointless and without benefit of any kind. If your partner tries to engage you forcefully, seeking to show off his combative power, then I'll just use light and easy hand work to play around with him. Don't bother taking him seriously. If he cheats or acts disrespectfully, grabbing me wildly or jamming into me pointlessly then I'll change it over to free sparring; ratcheting up in this way is a legitimate response when necessary. When you switch over to sparring, your body needs to move sinuously like a playful dragon, your spirit like a wild horse, so that the slightest motion of your internal energy shoots straight into his body. If you try to rely on flaccid half-hearted actions you'll never defeat a really skilled fighter. You must be able to change suddenly, hit instantaneously, and generally act with extreme speed and precision. Your spirit must combust inside and emerge with shocking power like thunder that overwhelms him with shock and awe. This is the only correct way.

There are only five basic tastes [in TCM], but in practice flavours are infinite. There are only five basic tones in the [traditional pentatonic] scale, but variations and combinations of these are infinite. The Art of War [Sun-zi] has only 13 chapters yet its applications in real situations are beyond count. Similarly, Taijiquan has only thirteen basic movements [postures] yet the art is absolutely inexhaustible.

The slowness and softness of Taiji practice are intended to cultivate perceptual sensitivity, to temper and maximize the spirit energy, and to clarify the mind. Your responses must be so deftly sensitive and your issuing of energy tightly focused into any opening that you can sense. The energy emerges suddenly and abruptly penetrates anywhere that he can't defend - that's how four ounces defeats a thousand pounds. This is the most sophisticated form of offensive fighting.

If your spirit energy is insufficient, or your perceptual abilities are inadequate, then your opponent will feel your energy before it can be issued, and though it may be strong you won't be able to apply it. You full power can only manifest if you're sensitive enough to perceive everything about him while keeping your own power hidden, your issuance of energy will be fast and fully effective.

I have an opinion about the current generation of Taijiquan teacher that can be summarized as follows: many of them have an understanding of the soft skill and relaxed power. However, their embodiment of the power of lively emptiness is still insufficient, not adequately refined.

Therefore, though a given teacher's skill may be great, but since his understanding of lively emptiness falls short, his internal energy therefore remains sub-par. Zheng Manqing (Cheng Man Ching) had a true appreciation of lively emptiness and his skilfulness has been witnessed many times.

My Students Don't Want To Do Push Hands

I've heard this said, yet if push-hands is an integral part of tai chi what is it that has been putting them off the idea, until now? In previous newsletters I've discussed the power of words as 'the word is not the thing' so in this situation, another aspect to consider is relevance and/or context. When push-hands is only considered from one perspective then maybe it doesn't seem relevant or even appropriate so I thought I would discuss some of the many and varied facets of push-hands to enable connection to a wider purpose and thereby find relevance.

Often the term 'pushing hands' is taken literally with the intention outward and forward, pushing and shoving, whilst trying to grab onto the ground in some sort of egocentric challenge. Yet a more descriptive term would be 'sensing hands' where the aims are:

To develop sensory acuity
To connect with your partner
To connect to the ground
To connect to the flow of energy of interaction
To blend, neutralise and redirect

With this in mind, let's look at some potential applications of push-hands (Tui Shou). The first and most obvious is the martial application of off-balancing and uprooting you opponent. The next is the polar opposite where the aim is to sense imbalance in a person with the aim of rebalancing them to the point that they feel more stable and safe. Jenny said there is a more obvious application of being close enough to have a chat about what was on TV last night whilst attempting some sort of partner dance that sneaks under the teacher's radar.

The first part of push-hands should actually be called connecting-hands as the aim is to meet and connect with your partner/opponent. The next stage is to connect the energy pathway to the ground or to become aware/attuned to the energy pathway to the ground. The final stage is application. Regardless of your use of push-hands, only the final stage changes as this is the stage of application or usage of the energies developed/refined within push-hands and in-turn tai chi practice in general. Mindful practice of application is essential.

The main failing in push-hands is the initial connection intention (or purpose of connection intention). By connecting with the intention "I reach out and connect with you to develop kinaesthetic awareness, of who and where we are in space. To develop proprioception" we connect to our own balance and awareness. This sensory acuity (calibration) is key to our development whatever the end goal.
Application comes from mindful connection with purpose; it doesn't matter whether you intend to off-balance or re-balanced the connection stage is the same.
Reach out and connect to your partner; take that connection and connect it to the ground. Next neutralise, redirect and apply. Neutralise means 'take to neutral' it does not mean run away from or resist. For the pusher it may initially feel as if they could still push yet they are not able to direct the force without losing balance. At the next level the pusher will feel as if they are falling into emptiness which is the stage at which they lose their connection to the ground. The next stage is where you either choose to accelerate them into a waiting wall or rebalance them into safe stability.
So back to the question of why bother with push-hands. The simple rule is "to off-balance, don't let your opponent connect to the ground" or "to re-balance, reconnect your partner to the ground". This disconnection or connection creates either panic or peace of mind so next time you consider how to present push-hands ask yourself "what is the purpose?" because it is an amazing practice tool that can both harm or heal; I should know, I've used it for both.

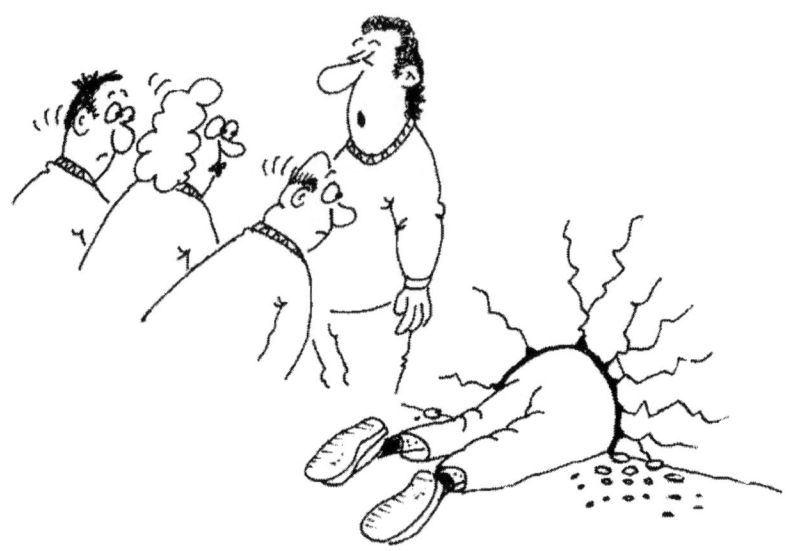

A point to Reflect on

Why practice partner work, I'm not interested in the 'martial' aspects of Taiji?

Fighting is fighting however you paint it, but partner work is more about knowing yourself than anything else. There are many aspects of personal contact and human interrelations to explore but my focus hear will be on mental and physical balance. I have said before that root and balance are a product of relaxation and the natural effects of gravity; the question here may be how we know we are relaxed and aligned. Simple, you stop falling over and start falling though your body.

Partner work here has the instant awareness of errors in ourselves. Right now you weight an amount, same as you will by the end of the day and most likely same as you did yesterday. The fact is we are less aware of errors as we are comfortable in ourselves; but if a partner adds a little pressure or you pick up a heavy item, you become instantly aware you knees or back etc. are strained (not relaxed). You could wait years to find this small error that adds up to cause serious problems, or you can find it now and fix it; I know which I'd prefer....

Ben Lo said you have to suffer a little pain in your youth to aid a pain free old age, by which he meant work hard now to invest in your future.

Here we have the chance to develop and improve our awareness and physical balance, to 'invest in our future'. By practicing push-hands we have the chance to appreciate errors in our movement, feel our axis, connect to the ground and allow compression (pung) to naturally occur. With a little outside pressure during form practice we can slowly eradicate errors in transitional movements; are you hips level, is you lower back tense? Could they be better? Ask you partner for feedback...

To invest in loss, to relax our mind and explore what is happening within our minds and bodies, as we flow though life is an extraordinary feeling. To live in the 'here and now' is an opportunity not to be missed. Ask you instructor to explain yielding, which by the way is not running away, and get a sense of meeting a force in a way that puts you into balance but does not feel like resistance. Tai Chi is a wondrous art that could be called 'body balance' or body/mind work but they do not quite have the same mystical appeal...

The true benefits of partner work are increased awareness of the here and now; of whom and where we are and our relationship to the world and everything around us.

Of course it has a martial benefit but that is superficial compared to that mentioned above.

Hands— The Fine Tools Of Internal Arts

Our hands sense and send messages to the brain to be interpreted, but they also need to be able to emit a powerful force. There are up to 21,000 sensors of heat, pressure, and pain per square inch in the fingertips alone.

One sixth of all the body's muscles are devoted to hand movements. A single hand movement can involve as many as 50 muscles working together.

They are 'the fine' that need to be taken care of, and they will serve you well over a lifetime

Next time you do push hands give a thought to this and what is actually going on as you touch.

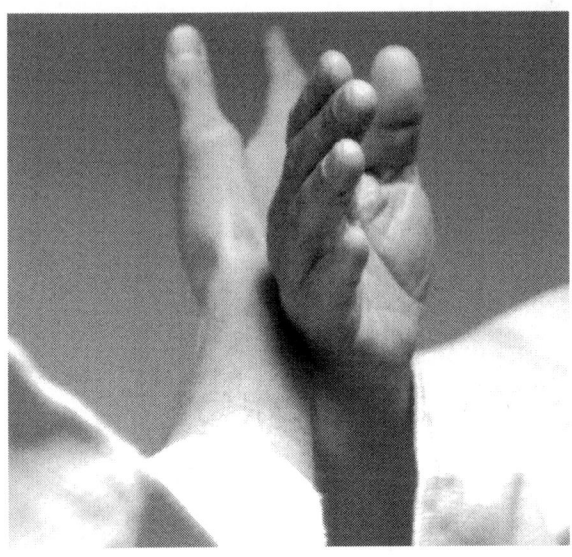

Energy Forward Corresponding Movement Backward

Boats do not have brakes so as they move towards the dock they have to put their engines into reverse to slow it down; push-hands applies same principle and only comes with practice yet it is often overlooked. I hope you all remember the 5 steps of "left to go right, right to go left, up to go down, down to go up and centre". Let's consider them with a new perspective of working together rather than 'this then that' or backwards to go forwards. When I was first taught the concept of the 5 steps I was told "if you want to uproot somebody then as they push you, let go then push them – backwards to go forwards". This works fine on beginners over over-enthusiastic combatants (oops partners) but rarely on anyone with any sensitivity. Next you can play with the idea of making space to re-attack or "get out of the way so you can have another go" – left to go right – step off to the left and re-enter to attack after they've missed.

I'd like to take it further, as the example given by the boat coming into port, and consider both directions working together as in 'step back to repulse the monkey' or rollback with forward intention/expansion. When pushing to uproot somebody, if your push is only in one direction, forwards, then it is easy to overrun and be uprooted yourself; this reverse movement is experienced in Huang's 5th loosening exercise. When moving left to go right, or right to go left, both directions work together not separately to sever the root of your opponent/partner; this action is referred to as 'split' (Li) and is one of the 8 energies. Applying split prevents your partner from connecting to your single direction of energy by not having a single direction of energy; this is yin-yang in action as the interaction is always flowing. Next time you practice ward-off left look for the flow of 'left to go right' then start to look to each posture to find the flow of corresponding movements before applying it in the live field we call push-hands.

Chinese Character Yan (Ren)

The Chinese character Yan is formed by combining two Chinese characters, that is, the word for knife and the word for heart. The top character of Yan (Ren) is that of knife while the bottom character Xin is that of heart.

$$刃_{REN} + 心_{XIN} = 忍_{REN}$$
(Blade of the knife) (Heart) (Patience)

The Chinese word Yan (Ren) denotes patience and tolerance. This character is often found in many Martial Arts Schools. To truly understand the meaning of this character, there is a proverb that is said with the character which conveys its essence:

"YAN YUT SEE, FUNG PENG
LONG ZHENG.
TUI YUT BOW, HOI FOOT
TIEN HOUNG".
(Cantonese Language)

If one is patient and tolerant for a time,
The winds will even and waves will calm
If one gives way,
Skies will clear and seas will widen for you.

Having patience also means having the qualities of quiet steady perseverance. You must have steady persistence in your course of action when met with obstacles, challenges and discouragement. Only then will you keep going to meet success.

Part 2 - Meditation & Mindfulness

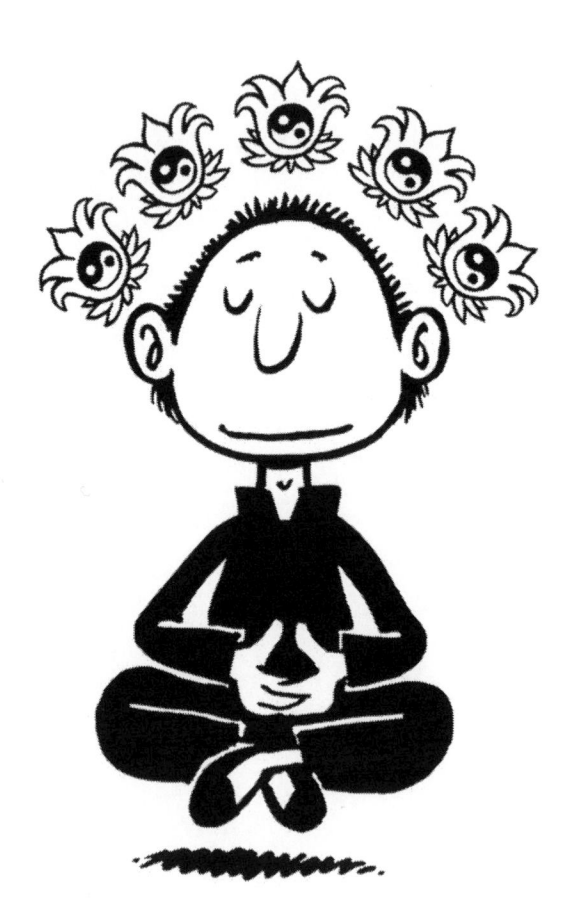

The Mindfulness of Tai Chi Chuan
Mindfulness is the miracle which calls back in a flash our dispersed mind and restores it to wholeness so that we can live each moment of life.

A Meditation For You To Try

*** The Pebble....

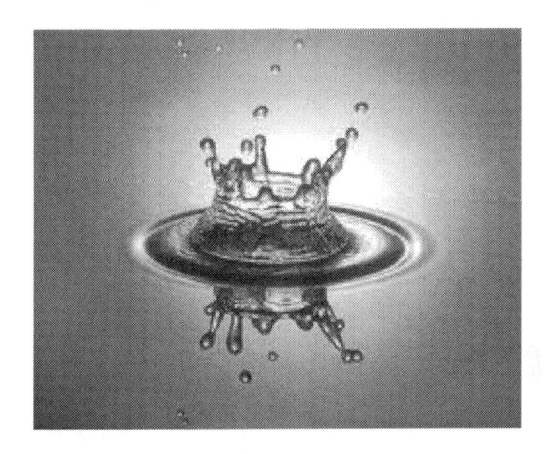

While sitting still and breathing slowly, think of yourself as a pebble which is falling through a clear stream.

While sinking, there is no intention to guide your movement.

Sink toward the spot of total rest on the gentle sand of the riverbed.

Continue meditating on the pebble until your mind and body are at complete rest:
A pebble resting on the sand.

Maintain this peace and relaxation for a half hour while watching your breath.

No thoughts about the past or future can pull you away from your present peace.
The universe exists in this present moment.

No desire can pull you away from this present peace.

There are many many meditations, so if you have a favourite that maybe is not so well publicized let us have it and we can put it in our next book to share with others.

On Teaching

No man can reveal to you aught but that which already lies half asleep in the dawning of our knowledge.
The teacher who walks in the shadow of the temple, among his followers , gives not of his wisdom but rather of his faith and his lovingness.

If he is indeed wise he does not bid you enter the house of HIS wisdom, but rather leads you to the threshold of YOUR OWN mind.
The astronomer may speak to you of his understanding of space, but he cannot give you HIS understanding.
The musician may sing to you of the rhythm which is in space, but he cannot GIVE you the ear which arrests the rhythm, nor the voice that echoes it.
And he who is versed in the science of numbers can tell of the regions of weight and measure, but he cannot conduct YOU thither.
For the vision of one man lends not its wings to another man.

Taken from THE PROPHET by KAHLIL GIBRAN

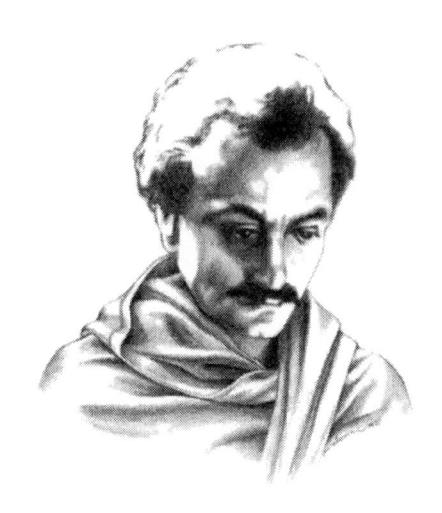

The Miracle of Mindfulness

Mindfulness is the miracle which calls back in a flash our dispersed mind and restores it to wholeness so that we can live each moment of life.

I was given a book recently by a friend that made me reconsider my focus a little. The book was called 'the miracle of mindfulness' and is a Zen manual for meditation. As I read and digested each page it reminded me of a Chinese proverb we've spoken of before, 'neglecting the near in search of the far'; but more than this it tells us to focus on each instant and enjoy its detail. I will quote the Sutra of mindfulness and go from there:

When walking, the practitioner must be conscious that he is walking. When sitting, the practitioner must be conscious that he is sitting. When lying down, the practitioner must be conscious that he is lying down..... No matter what position one's body is in, the practitioner must be conscious of that position, Practising thus, the practitioner lives in direct and constant mindfulness of the body...

Over the next few weeks just try and pay attention to the instant you are in and experience it.

My aim is not to go all 'new-age' on you; it is to highlight the importance of mind and body as one. We are a collection of learnt experiences but we generally do not choose how to experience the experiences, rather we let them happen to us. Maybe you've heard somebody say *"They always get themselves into a terrible state"* but what does this really mean? To learn more efficiently to be in control of the state we are in, we need to pay close attention to the moment we are in and build a sort of calibrated scale of feeling and experience. Why muddle through for years and years making slow progress.
The old Chinese saying of *'We must learn to taste bitter before we can taste sweet'*

is very wise; it doesn't say how much bitter or for how long.... Did you know our brains are programmed to see the negative before the positive in everything? This is essential to our fight or flight response. To learn, be mindful of your response so it can be learnt more quickly and allowed to develop into an unconscious action. Through mindful practice, notice the natural change from bitter to sweet and feel the feeling.....

Tai Chi is an art of change, ever evolving and moving with the flow of life, not standing still or stagnating; embrace this change. When you are aware and accept that everything around you is constantly changing, and that you have no control over 99% of it, you are able to embrace change like a close friend! Change is a like a river, constantly flowing and moving things around. The river of life is constantly bringing you ideas, people, situations – each one is an opportunity to be enriched or to enrich others, and to learn.

Try and focus on developing a natural root and 'whole body movement', not just in one direction but all directions, walking through some of the postures like lotus kick to pay attention to the potential of each step. To be aware that all parts are alive and vital, one must be mindful of the whole. Push hands is an act of non-resistance, of blending with all around you, and so is the form. To bask in each moment is the true glory of Tai Chi, to be aware of yourself and all around you will show you the wonders that life has to offer. But before you all start to run screaming "**Mad hippy**", know that Tai Chi is truly a martial art of amazing refinement, able to offer each of you with the patience, great rewards.

An Introduction to Meditation

The words 'meditation' and 'mindfulness' have become commonplace in today's culture. In the world of counselling and psychotherapy there are constant references to mindfulness and within various spiritual circles, particularly Buddhism, and others that some might call the 'new-age', meditation is a common practice for achieving many psychological 'states'. It has been around for a long time. I first came across Zen meditation as a student while studying Karate. Later, as I trained as a Psychotherapist, I came to appreciate the wide ranging benefits of the practise to many aspects of my clients psychological health by helping people relax, manage disturbing emotions, cope with trauma memories and more. I then did some courses in Buddhist Psychology and Meditation and then, it goes without saying, I found Tai chi!

This is the first of several articles exploring different aspects of meditation. I wish to generally orientate the reader and offer some initial suggestions as to how to make a start in what, if you take it seriously, will become a lifelong endeavour not dissimilar to our art of Tai Chi.

To some people meditation is mistakenly believed to mean a cutting off all detachment from ordinary concerns however nothing could be further from the truth. Meditation is in fact the focused awareness on what 'is', the 'present moment', and there are many different methods to achieve this.

Perhaps it would be most appropriate to start with a basic introduction to two of the main types of meditation. The first is known as 'concentration' or in Sanskrit 'Samadhi'. The second is known as 'insight' meditation, in Sanskrit, 'Vipassana'.

'Concentration' meditation consists of many techniques evolved in different cultures. It is used to enable a person to concentrate their awareness sometimes using an external object such as a flame, a flower or other imagined objects such as a cloud or anything of the person's choice. Of the many methods available perhaps the most common is the 'mindfulness of breathing' which is what I will introduce later on in this article.

The other form of meditation known as 'insight' oriented meditation is usually embarked upon once a person has achieved a satisfactory ability in the former. Within this, one meditates on various problems, metaphors or prescribed visualisations. Two classic examples of these are the 'Koans' one often finds in Zen – "Does a dog have Buddha nature?" and certain visualisations that one finds in the Tibetan Tantric traditions – for example, imaging a connection with the deity Manjushri via the breath and crown chakra. In fact Gautama Buddha would prescribe various visualisations to fit the different temperaments and the elements of the person he was offering it to. One could almost say this may have been an early form of psychotherapy for people who were perhaps obsessional, lazy, over committed, anxious, depressed, stressed etc.

There is nothing wrong with engaging in some of these practices along with basic concentration, in fact in the Zen tradition it is argued that sudden 'awakening' – (the spiritual aim of meditation) can occur at any time without the years of preparation and practice.

A checklist for your meditation posture

This checklist will allow you to run through a quick routine to allow for optimal performance in meditation.

1. Adjust your seat height and angle so that your back is relatively straight, and also relaxed.
2. Make sure that your hands are supported so that there's no strain in your shoulders or between the shoulder-blades.
3. Relax your shoulders, letting them roll back to open your chest. Let your shoulders move with your breathing.
4. Take a few deep breaths into the upper chest to allow your chest to open. Relax on the out-breath, but see if you can keep a sense of space across the front of the chest.

5. Adjust the angle of your head, so that the back of your neck is relaxed, long and open, and your chin is slightly tucked in.
6. Relax your jaw, your tongue, your eyes and your brow.

The following meditation is taught by the FWBO: 'Friends of the Western Buddhist Order' and is a simple introductory meditation to enable us to experience the initial stages of meditation – quieting the mind. It starts with some guidance with regards to posture

The Practice
The mindfulness of breathing we give the breath our full attention. We use the physical sensations of the breath as an object that we focus on. We just allow the breath to happen. This is not a breathing exercise. We simply observe, and see what happens.
Stage 1 Count 1-10 just after each out breath (breath 1, breath 2 etc)
Stage 2 Count 1-10 just before each in breath (1 breath, 2 breath etc)
Stage 3 Stop counting and experience the general flow of the breath
Stage 4 Maintain your attention at the point where you are most aware of the breath e.g. your nostrils, lips or perhaps your belly.

Our Tai Chi form has sometimes been called 'meditation in movement' and then we think about the ebb and flow, expansion and contraction, expand and release, so beautifully demonstrated in our art, we can think that with our breathing and right focus it is indeed meditation in movement.

Furthermore when we think about our Qigong sets, the first principle is 'structural alignment', the second is 'breath' and the third is our 'attention and intention', hence, we shouldn't be thinking about work or what we are going to do when the session ends – we should be either 'empty' (as far as possible) or visualising according to the prescriptions of the form. An example would be the 'microcosmic orbit' during standing post. The same three principles occur in any good meditation.

Later in the book, I'll discuss the 'point' of meditation, psychological, spiritual or physical? Or all three? Some history of the different aspects Buddhism and Daoism and how meditation practices have been influenced by these, and finally, offer some more suggestions for practice.

> *Blessed are the Flexible*
> *For we shall not*
> *Be bent out of shape*

Stillness

We have always found that a large majority of students of Tai Chi begin attending classes for the purpose of the health benefits of the relaxation and focus that is at the core of the art.
We drag along all the days stresses from our work, or problems at home and at times the weight that everyday life sometimes puts on our "tense" shoulders.
I know that when I have a "bad" day and I feel as though I am in "5th gear", which for me means racing round but getting nothing done, I have to take a moment to put on "the brakes and change down."
I think maybe we should think about this as applied within the weekly Tai Chi class.
Some of us rush in late so already we are still in top gear before we commence, some get there early to practice before the class begins, either way everyone starts the warm up still with the shoulders physically up and the mind psychologically "up".

Why not get to the training venue 5 or 10 minutes early and just "be".
Stand with eyes closed (if it helps) bring down your breaths to a comfortable level and begin working your way around the muscles in your body, from the feet up or the head down, doesn't really matter, just focus on any tension you find and let it go as you breathe out.
Feel right to your fingertips and toes, hopefully as you progress you will be surprised at how warm they can become as the tension leaves.
When you have worked your way round the outside of the body, the oxygen to the brain (mind) should be improved by the muscles relaxing and allowing the blood in the veins to flow more freely.
Major organs will also benefit from this and their function should improve.
You will be surprised how much better your focus will be once the class officially begins.
You will hopefully with regular practice be able to change out of 5th gear and begin your class in 'neutral'

Give this some thought; it could add a whole new dimension to your practice.
You can practice this anytime.....

In the BOOK OF 5000 WORDS which is attributed to Lao Tse the great Taoist scholar, it is *written "The substantial is the root of the insubstantial; the STILL is the master of what moves"* (inner calm)

I find it really hard to meditate in what some may call the traditional way, but find this exercise helps lead my mind into a more peaceful place and helps to bring my shoulders 'down'.
Learn to *Jing Zhou* – "sit quietly".

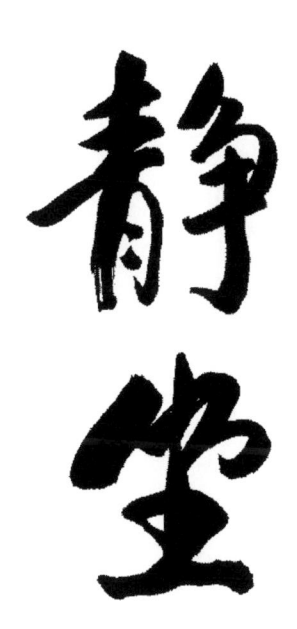

静坐

Meditation part 2

Following on from Part 1, earlier in this chapter, I would like to discuss some of the most common difficulties people have when starting a formal meditation practice. In future articles I will explore some of the spiritual systems underpinning the practice (Buddhist, Daoist, Hindu) and their links with Qigong, (Neigong), Tai chi and Martial Arts in general. Before that however, it is really worth 'getting a feel' for the practice.

So, after you have spent time finding an appropriate place to sit, organising your time, buying some incense, set up a shrine and told the family (all optional – you really can do it anywhere with no special objects – but sometimes a little ritual helps!) then it is time to actually just do it!

It is at this stage that we start to experience the physical discomfort, the wandering 'monkey' mind, shopping lists, previous hurts, future fantasies etc.

A long time ago, the Buddhists outlined a helpful system for understanding and working with these phenomena, collectively known as the 'hindrances'.

They are grouped in to five:
1. Desire for sense experience (Craving):- food, sex etc
2. Sloth and Torpor:- sleepiness, heaviness, can't be bothered…
3. Doubt and Indecision:- Sceptical, doubt regarding ability…
4. Ill Will:- Irritation, anger, hatred.
5. Restlessness and Anxiety:- Physical inability to settle, mental worry…

We all experience these from time to time, sometimes we just can't let go of something, can't relax, sometimes we fall asleep, sometimes we keep being distracted by cars or coughs or other people shuffling. One needs commitment and perseverance! It helps to have a 'point' – a reason for doing it and we'll discuss how complex and paradoxical this is in a future article.

Meanwhile, there are 'antidotes' to these 'hindrances'. However, ideally, you would undertake a 'course' or an apprenticeship and work for many years on these as one is never truly 'free' of them. Even if you attained 'enlightenment' (a Buddhist concept and aim of meditation if done for spiritual development) you would still have a physical body to work with, relationships to manage and washing up to do!

This is summed up in a wonderful book entitled 'After the Ecstasy, the Laundry' by Jack Kornfield – and Buddhist Psychologist and teacher.

The antidotes are:

1. **Awareness** – Noticing the problem/hindrance, acknowledging it.
2. **Sky like attitude** – Allowing your awareness to be bigger than the hindrance so that it just fades or passes by (like a cloud).
3. **Cultivating the opposite** – compassion to challenge ill will, resolve and commitment to challenge doubt and indecision.
4. **Consider the consequences**.

Inner Peace: This is so true

If you can start the day without caffeine,
If you can be cheerful, ignoring aches and pains,
If you can resist complaining and boring people with your troubles,
If you can eat the same food every day and be grateful for it,
If you can understand when you're loved ones are too busy to give you any time,
If you can take criticism and blame without resentment,
If you can conquer tension without medical help,
If you can relax without alcohol,
If you can sleep without the aid of drugs,

　...Then, You Are Probably .... the family dog

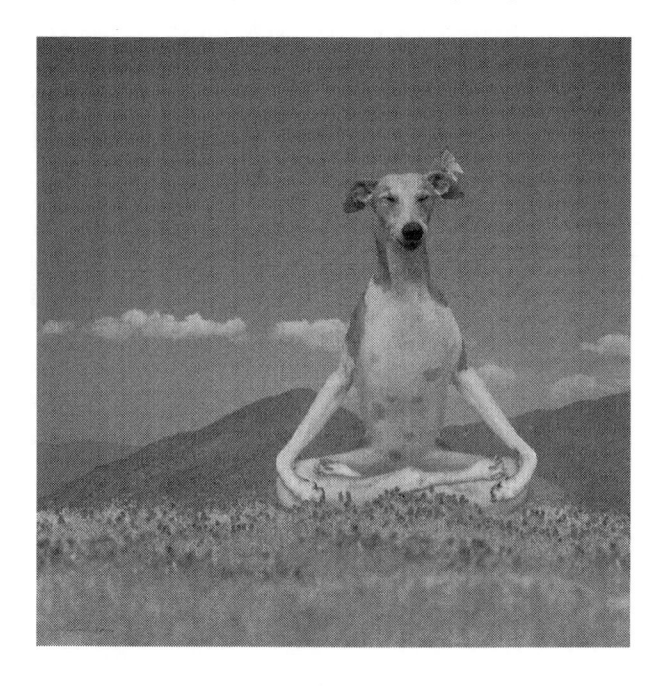

Chinese Proverbs - The Chinese Puzzle Unravelled
(A Little!)

We all have read little books of proverbs, be they Western or Eastern and marvelled at how simple things around us are explained and really many cultures can overlap in their thoughts and daily life.
The problem we have with Chinese proverbs and sayings is that many in classical books are quotes from even earlier sages and therefore may appear as anonymous or traditional.

This practice continues but it is the quote not the author which is important.
Deng Xiaoping once said: "What matter if a cat is black or white, so long as it catches mice!" Even this offering was an age old saying!
There was a cluster of proverbs in a brief era around 2,500 years ago in late Zhou Dynasty.
It was around this era that Lao Zi, Confucius (Kong Qui) and Mencius (Meng Zi)
There were many followers of these great sages and people where considered uneducated if they could not digest and regurgitate the words of the classics.

Strangely enough although there are thousands of quotes, sayings, and proverbs they probably all come from just a handful of wise men, handed down and scattered as leaves in the wind to many who repeated them.
These saying can be found in songs, poems, and some just used in general Chinese conversation.
The Book of Songs has hundreds of ancient poems mostly listed as anonymous.
The Imperial Yue-fu (or music bureau) kept records of the most popular to keep the Emperor informed of the general mood of the country.
A proverb may also derive its origin from an ancient piece of folklore, often based on some long forgotten event. Some of these can be found in the popular Chinese fortune cookie.

Emperor Qin Shi Huang-di 221 BC, mainly known for the Terracotta Warriors that guard his grave, was tyrannical as a ruler and burned most of the books around at the time he was in power to discourage any debate.
Few survived, the classics, including Confucius and the Book of Changes, are among the few that where left to us.

We can all find humour and inspiration in the sage's words and they cover most areas of life and living. They are deep, profound and often very beautifully written.
Many of the poems and proverbs take on a different meaning when we discover that the WILD GOOSE is a symbol of letters and communication, and "TRAPPED AMONG FLOWERS" is to fall in love. "SPRING" the season, also means youth and, in some cases, stirrings of love.
The most innocent of verses takes on an extra salacious dimension when we understand that to "MAKE THE RAIN AND CLOUDS" is to make love, and that the Chinese characters for "WOMAN" and "EYEBROW" combine to mean "flirt"

This quote attributed to Chairman Mao is sadly still quite relevant today in some countries, so I will end with it
"Political power grows out of the barrel of a gun"

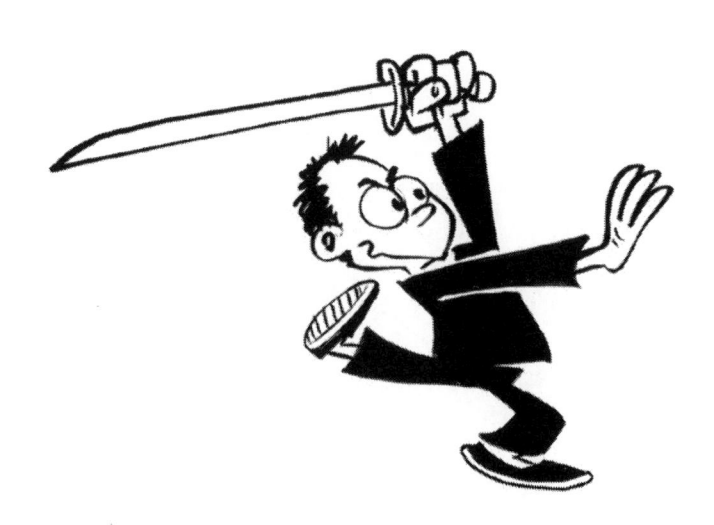

Movement and stillness conspired one day

Movement and stillness conspired one day. Movement said "I am life. The constant changing of the sea, the rustle of the wind, the scampering of the lizard on the rock."
Stillness said nothing
Movement went on, "Everything that lives, moves. Life itself is movement and change-growing, running, slinking, dancing..."
Finally stillness answered, "at the bottom, your sea is deep and silent; your wind dances and then returns to calm; the scampering lizard issues from an egg containing its life and essence."
Movement thought for a while then added, "Thank you for teaching me. I see another viewpoint now. But you have to admit, you were forced to speak or I could not know."
Stillness nodded. And from that day they agreed to share equally the secrets of life.
Explore the internal environment, and not be overwhelmed by the external, enables the warrior to look to their stores of energy; to recuperate to regenerate. Without this stillness how can they know they are able to go on? Stillness unifies.

Movement creates punching and kicking, stillness creates root and patience. There are many methods of creating strength and stamina – running, weights, squats, but only one to gain a root.... Stillness.... Stillness practicing by just standing and being present, by sinking and connecting through present awareness.

Standing (Zhan Zhuang) is an integral part of tai chi and is more than just standing in the postures, it is about gaining stillness. Through it we develop strength, calm and even self-knowledge. The muscles ache, the body craves movement, the mind is beset by a 1000 fleeting thoughts – you itch, you remember a bill to pay, you become angry.

EXAMINES WELLBEING ARISING FROM 5 MINUTES OF STATIC CHI KUNG

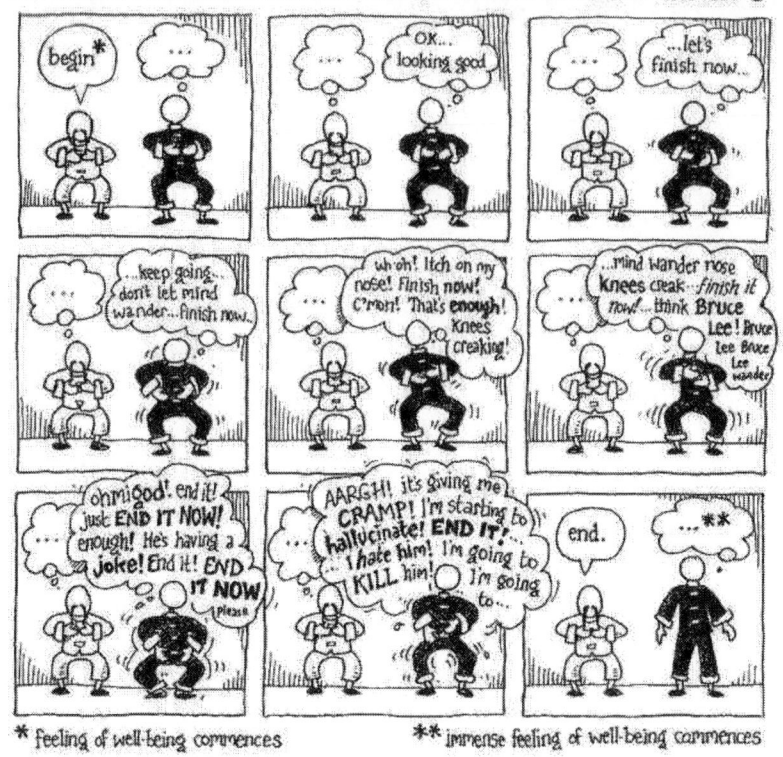

* feeling of well-being commences　　** immense feeling of well-being commences

Slowly, this dissolves into a world of attention that draws you into a universe of your own mind and body. After a while, you will have to face the fact that it is stillness itself you are fighting. "RELAX!" you cry! As the aches and thoughts try to seduce you away from calmness. "Mindfulness is wonderful; you just have to pay attention." To be present, to be still, takes practice as we have all been seduced by the wonders of noise and activity.

Stillness will enable you to develop into a ***Peaceful Warrior*** and you will find that things that bothered you previously no longer get quite the same reaction. The next time you take that first deep breath, get in position and stand still, searching for stillness, and consider the journey of self-discover found without even moving. Next time you feel you have lost your root, realise it is movement that stole it from you and stillness that will return it.

How To Get The Best From Your Brain

DAYDREAMING rests parts of the brain that do analytical or repetitive work. Indulging in daydreaming at least ten times a day gives you a chance to integrate your thoughts.

SEEK OUT SILENCE. At least ten minutes of silence a day gives your brain a break from its normal non-stop activity. Claude Debussy said: "Music is the silence between the notes."

TELL and be told stories. They are great for your creative imagination.

IMPROVE your social intelligence by asking and learning to listen.

Oh... to sit quietly

I would love to sit quietly, but the world is such a noisy place
As I still my mind the world screams "listen to me"

As I strive for peace, the world nudges me
As I try to shut it all out, the world bags on the door.

Oh how I wish all could be quiet so I could just sit quietly
But as I do I realise the beauty of it all
The beauty of the flow of life…

Maybe if I stopped resisting life and flowed with it
I could enjoy the peace within the noise and just sit quietly.....

Breathing And The Mind

I always begin my Tai Chi practice with a deep exhalation, to remove the carbon dioxide from the lungs, clear away scattered thoughts from the mind.

A gentle inhalation takes place, awareness increases, fingers are energized, palms are raised upward and outward, until a Tai Chi posture is formed.

The mind is fully awake and the lungs are filled with oxygen.
When the lungs need to release carbon dioxide, exhalation naturally follows.

With a slow deflation of energy, the palms gradually fall downward and move inward.

Expel all wasted air and all anxious thoughts are reduced, my hips are relaxed again and the posture is dissolved. There is plenty of room for incoming oxygen after slow and long inhalations. The slow motion practice of Tai Chi Chuan gives us a sufficient supply of oxygen for all body cell needs.
When we are happy, we inhale, the upper torso straightens when we are cheerful.

When we are unhappy, we exhale and our body sags.
The mind, body and breathing interact together.
When the mind begins to think, we inhale. Mind and body energize each other as active thoughts cause mind and body movements.

These are natural interactions. Breathing regulates the thought and alertness of the mind. Inhalation will increase thoughts or awareness in the mind, and exhalation help reduce the thoughts and awareness decreases.

The alertness and awareness pattern changes while a person is in deep sleep, when he takes in oxygen, it helps increase the awareness or stimulate alertness, as we exhale, we are less aware and alert.

Therefore, breathing and awareness and physical movements correspond to each other.

Taken from –Breathing and Awareness of the Mind by William CC Chen.

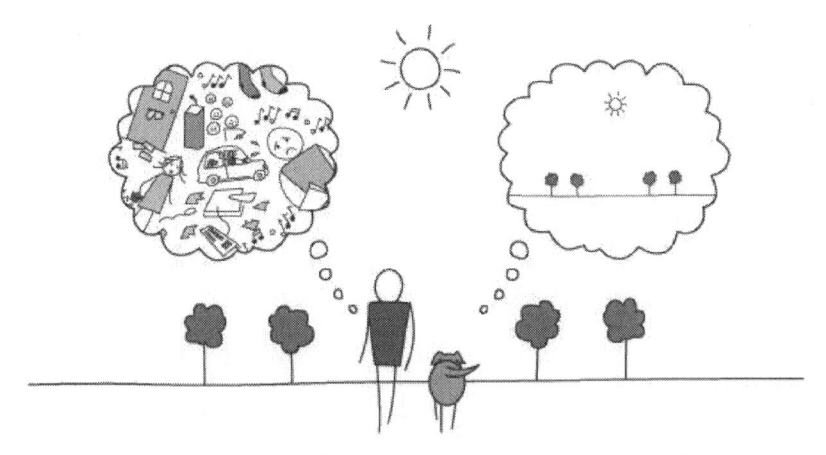

Mind Full, or Mindful?

Believe Nothing

A thought for the day

It is much easier to believe that it's snowing, than to experience the snow. If you just believe, you can stay inside, stay warm and avoid the cold. That's why people are led up the garden path by others beliefs. It's easier and warmer. And all this 'believing stuff' starts in kinder garden. In the context of your spiritual or personal growth, believe nothing, experiment and test everything, in the laboratory of your own experience. Only then will you be able to separate truth from falsehood, reality from illusion, and lead others with integrity. Challenge and check at least one belief every day.
And if it's found wanting, chuck it or change it. Challenge, check, then chuck or change, now that's a master at work.

Part 3 – Health

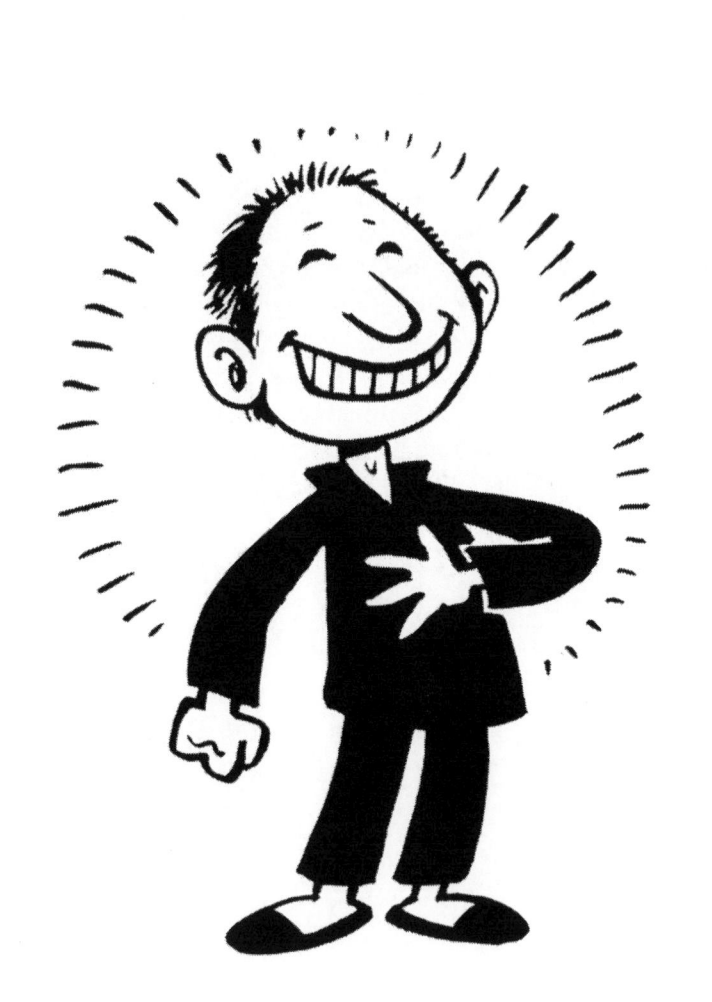

Values.

Master Cheng was holding a one-man show in America, and a businessman came to see the exhibit.
There was a large painting of a turtle with a price tag of $20,000.
The businessman stood in front of it for a long time, seemingly transfixed.
The next day he returned and asked those in charge, "Is it possible to negotiate a discount?"
They answered "No", but after a few days when the show was over and the staff were busy wrapping things up, the rich man returned with money in hand wanting to purchase the painting.
Cheng informed him that no sales could be concluded after the end of the show.

When the businessman asked, "What is the reason?" Cheng replied, "You love your money, and I love my painting.
We each have different values, and there is no basis for exchange."
The wealthy business man left, very disappointed. Cheng threw back his head and laughing said, "You can spend a thousand dollars and earn it back, but once this painting is gone, it is gone forever."

He held onto his painting, until 1982, when after his death, his wife presented it to the Palace Museum in Taipei.

How To Be Happy In 18 Easy Steps

1. Realise that great love and great achievements involve great risk.
2. When you lose, don't lose the lesson.
3. Follow the 3 Rs: Respect for self, Respect for others, Responsibility for you actions.
4. Remember that not getting what you want is often a stroke of luck!
5. Learn the rules so you know how to break them properly!
6. Don't let a little dispute injure a great relationship.
7. When you make a mistake, move to correct it immediately.
8. Spend some time alone every day.
9. Open your arms to change but don't let go of your values.
10. Remember that silence is sometimes the best answer.
11. Live a good, honourable life. Then when you get older and think back, you'll enjoy it a second time.
12. A loving atmosphere at home is the foundation of your life.
13. In disagreements with loved ones, deal only with the current situation. Don't bring up the past.
14. Share your knowledge. It is a way to achieve immortality.
15. Be gentle with the earth.
16. Once a year, go somewhere you've never been before.
17. Remember that the best relationship is one in which your love for each other exceeds your need for each other.
18. Judge your success by what you had to give up in order to achieve it.

"Good Karma" advice for life by the Dalai Lama.

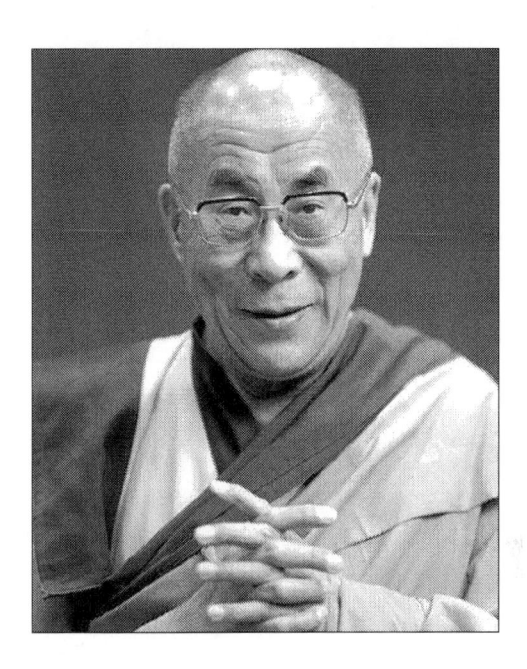

Maybe worth copying this out and putting it somewhere you will see it every day, or just taking a look when you feel the need to get back in touch with the truth.

Tai Chi Helps You Sleep Better.

Researchers report that practicing tai chi promotes sleep quality in older adults with moderate sleep complaints.
In a study, 112 healthy adults ranging in age from 59 to 86 were randomly assigned to one of two groups for a 25 week period:
The first group practiced 20 simple tai chi moves; the other participated in health education classes that included advice on stress management, diet and sleep habits.
At the beginning of the study, participants were asked to rate their sleep based on the Pittsburgh Sleep Quality Index, a self rated questionnaire that assesses sleep quality, duration and disturbances over a one month time interval.

The study found that the tai chi group showed improved sleep quality and a remission of clinical impairments, such as drowsiness during the day and inability to concentrate, compared with those receiving health education.
The tai chi participants showed improvements in their own self-rating of sleep quality, sleep duration and disturbance.

Taken from Autumn edition 2008 of the Tai Chi Chuan & Oriental Arts Magazine.

Preparing To Practice Qigong.

The Chinese traditional medical theory believes natural elements are vital supplements for your soul, spirit, and vigour.
Therefore sunny days and clear nights are recommended for your practice of Qigong as the preferred option.
Whilst inclement days of cloud, rain, or storms should be avoided.

Regulating the Position of the Body.
Sit down on a comfortable straight chair.
Make sure that your clothing is loose.
Relax completely. Draw in your shoulders slightly to relax your back.
Keep your head and neck in a straight line with your bottom.
Let your thighs and lower legs form a right angle.
Let your toes point in slightly towards each other, which makes your body into a circle.
Place your hands in your lap, palms upward, slightly touching your lower abdomen.
A male usually places his left hand on top of is right; a female places her right hand on top of her left one (but whichever feels the most comfortable for you is still fine)
Keep the thumb tips touching each other.
Relax your shoulders and elbows.
Touch your palate with your tongue.
Gently tighten your bottom.
Make sure that the top of your head (called the bai hui) is still in a straight vertical line with the centre of your bottom (called the hui ying).
Your body should be in perfect balance that you can easily maintain.
Let your eyes relax and lightly close.
Inhale and exhale naturally through your nose.
While inhaling, imagine your forehead cool and relaxed.
While exhaling, imagine all of your joints open and relax.
Whilst doing this exercise focus on the now, your existence and all the positive aspects of your being.
Be Mindful

Now continue....

Imagine that there is a stream of air that is flowing from your forehead through your face, your throat, your chest, and stomach.
Check your abdomen is relaxed and your bottom is still lightly tightened.
When the stream of air has reached the waist let it continue up your back to your shoulders, into your armpits, down to your elbows and wrists, until it reaches your fingertips.
Sit like this for a while.
When you feel ready to end this exercise, let your body relax as much as you can, let your arms hang loose at your side, feel the warmth spread down to the tips of your fingers.

Now commence the Qigong set you have chosen to do

This is a really nice practice to do before you start the day, or a great "time out" unwind evening session after a particularly stressful day.

A MOMENT.....

"And me, I still believe in paradise. But now at least I know it's not some place you can look for, cause it's not where you go. it's how you feel for a moment in your life, when you're a part of something, and if you find that moment….it lasts forever."

A line from the Movie "THE BEACH"

Talking Alignment. A Word From The Converted

Even as a trained nurse before I became a long time Tai Chi practitioner the words body alignment was just that, **WORDS**.

When you are feeling ok and have no muscular skeletal problems the necessity to invest in your body's future well-being may be far from your mind in this hectic life many of us lead.
From my first days in the hospitals school of nursing, the importance of correct lifting to protect our lower back was paramount.
We were warned of the risks of trying to move patients or lift them up the bed, or get them to their feet if they had fallen.
"Always make sure you work in two's" they told us
However on a ward at two o'clock in the morning when your colleague has gone for a break and a patient who is uncomfortable asks for help to change position, all that advice is forgotten in your desire to ease their discomfort.
Hence within the first 10 years of my career I developed a cervical spine (neck) problem, (confirmed by x-ray as mild degenerative changes) probably through patients putting their arm around it to get leverage up the bed, which at that time only gave me mild pain infrequently.
Little did I realise that my lumbar spine (lower back) was also silently suffering, with muscles struggling to compensate and relieve the pressure and minimise the problems I was creating for the future.
Things became worse with my cervical spine following the birth of my son (how does having a baby affect your neck you may ask!!!!!) Read on to find out…
Well meaning physiotherapists gave me the current advice for post natal women, which at that time was:-

To help involution of the uterus (in lay man's terms, flatten your stomach!) sleep on your stomach, with your head turned to one side, and as most of us have a favoured side which is more comfortable than the other, I put even more pressure on the muscles on my favoured side. (Many years later an osteopath could actually feel the tension in the affected side, and thought this may have helped the progression of my cervical degeneration which had been confirmed as now moderate, by x-ray.)

Too late, I have realised that there is no cure for this problem now (except in severe cases where operation may or may not help, and has its risks).

You can however reduce the times where nipping off the nerves that run through the vertebra occurs.

This can initiate their inflammation leading to pain and discomfort (headaches) for a few days until it settles on painkillers and anti-inflammatory medication.

These can in turn cause you other problems with your stomach etc. (the cure is sometimes as bad as the disease!)

I noticed that the day after I had been to a market or antique fair and therefore used my neck a lot turning to look side to side or up or down, I had an headache or at the very least a "muzzy" feeling all up the back of my neck into my head.

If my computer screen at work wasn't the right height, same thing.

Through Tai Chi I have learnt the words "correct alignment" and some years ago began using my waist to turn when I look back (instead of my neck to look over my shoulder etc) so now drop the hips turn from the waist has a NEW meaning, and has certainly decreased the episodes of discomfort I used to have which could last for a few days.

In fact the only times I get a "bad" recurrence is when I show beginners how **NOT** to perform a posture! without thinking of the consequence to myself until I am reminded the NEXT DAY.

My back pain is another story of self inflicted injury over a number of years, commencing I suppose insidiously with, yes, you guessed it, lifting patients badly.

Most nurses suffer the same problems, but I had to go one further didn't I!

In an effort to get fit and give up smoking (yes I know I should have known better than to start, no excuses) I started going to a gym and found myself "trapped" into high impact aerobics by a Jamie Curtis lookalike in a leotard that I couldn't decide whether she was trying to get into or out of as it fitted so tightly.
She assured me I to could have this figure within a few weeks of taking part in her class.
(I hasten to add this was well before my Tai Chi days)
As my abused lumbar spine had not yet really caused me any concern I was caught up in the heyday of gym mania.
Compounding the damage further to the music of "EYE OF THE TIGER" I cavorted around the studio punching the air, ducking and diving in the Boxacise Class.
Needless to say by the time I "found" Tai chi I had not achieved the desired shape, but I did have a lower back that meant if I stood too long it ached and I needed a cushion in the lumber area if I sat on a something that was too soft, my posture was bad and my poor muscles kept trying to pull together to align my spine that I had so stupidly neglected over the years.
I should have known better as a nurse, but eh nurses are human to and can be just as "blind" when it comes to thinking about accumulation of bad habits that are likely to give long term health issues.

Thanks to Tai Chi as with my neck, I am now consciously aware of keeping alignment from head to toe, so that my spine is not overloaded, or twisted, and that my muscles can slacken off a little and "enjoy" life as well!!!

It's never too late to work on your posture, and luckily within our Association a great deal of emphasis is put on this, and its benefits have been shown over and over again by student's improvements.
Jenny Peters SRN

How Tai Chi exercises benefit the knee joint

People will often blame the cause of their knee pain on arthritis rather than weakness or lack of stability in the joint itself. When we exercise, the body warms up and the joints release synovial fluid. Synovial fluid lubricates the joints of the body like engine oil does to various parts of a motor engine. As both the human body and a motor engine warm up their performance improves.

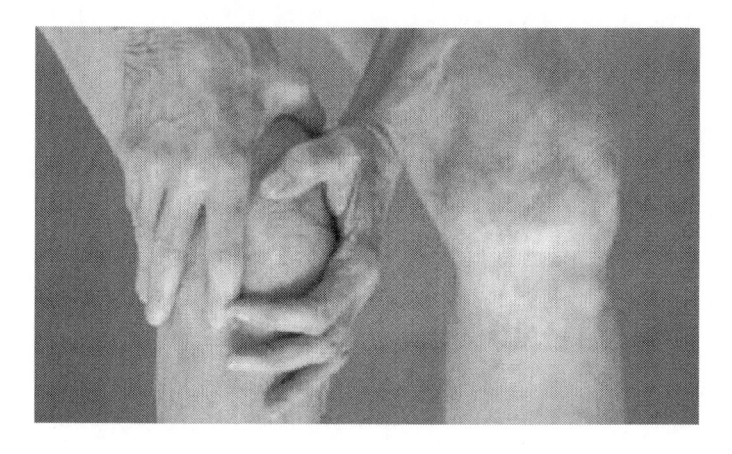

Most people who complain of knee pain will reduce their level of exercise to manage their pain. When in actual fact they should be doing gentle weight bearing exercise to increase the strength of their legs. This is where Tai Chi is beneficial. Tai Chi exercises increase the strength of the legs, increase synovial fluid production and reduce degeneration of the patella (knee cap). The quadriceps muscles on the front of the thigh, in particular vastus medialis (the tear drop shaped muscle on the inside line of the knee), play a key role in controlling the Q angle (the alignment) of the knee. If vastus medialis is weak and atrophied (muscle wastage) the knee cap becomes hyper mobile (moving around too much). This causes the head of the femur (thigh bone) to catch the back of the patella when climbing stairs or walking up and down hills. These factors increase the degeneration of the patella. The condition is known as chondra malacia patella (degeneration or softening of the knee cap) and causes considerable pain and discomfort.

By performing the Tai Chi warm up exercises, the Tai Chi form and especially Huang's five loosening exercises, the knee joints become more strong and stable. This, in turn, improves the student's performance, reduces their pain, and improves their quality of life.

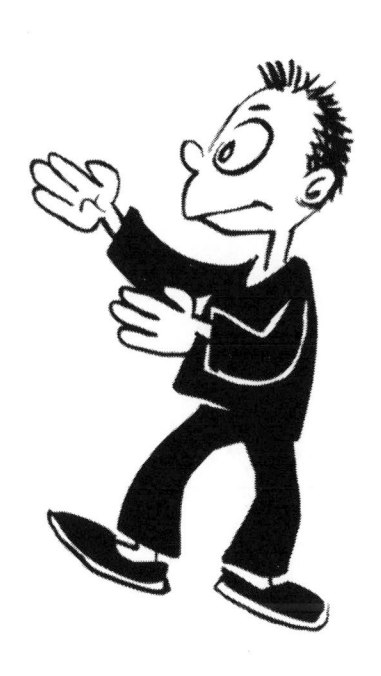

Qigong - Get Started.

The development of Qigong in China has been a very long and slow process.

Over a period of maybe three or four thousand years it has been gradually refined and technically adapted by practitioners who have learned from experience and guidance's of others, that the art can now be used as a wonderful aid to maintaining good health, physically and mentally throughout life.

It has also developed so well that it is a great add on to people who are already suffering from an established chronic disease and using prescription medication.

The belief in traditional Chinese medicine is that chronic illness is the result of "damage to the Severn Emotions"

In terms of Western medicine, these are stress-related diseases

It can help lift mood, help anxiety, increase oxygen intake by improving lung capacity thus aiding circulation and generally help give a feeling of well being.

In ancient times it was known as Dao Yin (which roughly can be translated as gymnastics). Tu Na (breath control) and Yang Sheng (body building).

Qigong has a long history of association with religious life in China, and the tradition suffered parallel divisions.

On the medical side, several distinct schools arose-Buddhist, Taoist, Confucian, and Wushu, along with a good many local styles stressing different technical variants etc.

All these styles are also found among China's minority peoples, and it has often been through these practitioners that Qigong methods and traditions have become established abroad, especially for instance in Japan. But now it has spread so far into the Western society that it is sometimes been called "WIGONG!"

Qigong has strongly influenced the development of Traditional Chinese Medicine, and indeed the impact has been reciprocal, in the present era, and especially since the seventies, the body of knowledge has undergone further refinement and its principles have been extended, not only in China where it originated, but also among an ever increasing worldwide body of experts, so that it has become a new kind of "science of well-being".

Qigong IS NOT A QUICK FIX it requires patient and diligent practice.
Below is an idea of what you can achieve health wise if like most things in life you are prepared to wait awhile

QIGONG timescale for improvement—

WITHIN 3 MONTHS—A general loosening up of the body and gradual feeling of improved well-being.
Shoulders and neck muscles relax off, and if you are prone to headaches these should lessen.
You may notice your back muscles, that have been tight and painful at times, (maybe through injury) now feel that they are beginning to be troublesome less often.

WITHIN 6 MONTHS—
You will suddenly be aware, because of the subtle, soothing, and exact movements of your daily practice, any aches and pains that where caused by bad posture will now be improving or gone.

1 YEAR—
You will experience less colds and viral infections, (there is evidence from research that practice of Tai Chi (which is a Qigong) boosts the immune system substantially.
Headaches vary rare or not at all.
Stamina has increased, and you will cope with the usually stresses and strains of life much more adequately.
Sleep improves and you will feel "more rested and refreshed" when you start the day.
You start to sense muscular tension at its onset and are able to consciously relax the parts of the body concerned.

There are many people who will attest to the general improvement in their health that they have experienced since becoming serious daily practitioners of this ancient art.
However as you all know "the proof of the pudding is in the eating".
Even if you can only fit in 10 minutes before or after work, "or maybe during a lunch break" get started.

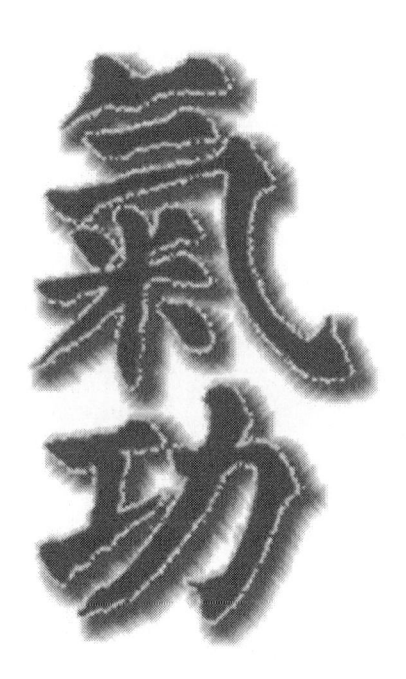

Before Tai Chi – By Ron Davies

I was asked to put down on paper my journey through ill health and the new beginning that I feel Tai Chi has bought me to.
I am no writer and it was a daunting task, but it was suggested maybe I would find diary form easier.

So here goes. ----
December 1999
I was taken to hospital as an emergency with chest pain, pain in my left arm and face, which was diagnosed as a major heart attack (coronary thrombosis) and it was so severe that I was immediately transferred to another local hospital that had facilities for performing heart bypass operations which it was felt I needed urgently to save my life.
Luckily the operation went well, and after discharge I was asked by the Physiotherapist to attend the hospital Gym once a week for 4 weeks for exercise classes to speed recovery.---------

April 2002
Referred to the hospital by my GP for abdominal pains.
Consultant felt the pain could be from my prostate gland, and that he needed to take a biopsy (a small piece of tissue from the gland) Unfortunately it turned out to be cancer of the Prostate and I faced another major operation, after which I felt very low and the only exercise I could do was aimed at my pelvic floor muscles to strengthen them.

JUNE 2004
Went through another bad time with my health, something was going on in my abdomen again. In and out of hospital with infections, even spent a few weeks on crutches! Because I found I couldn't walk properly because of them.
After another operation I spent a month in hospital on antibiotics and when I eventually returned home I was so low even thought I had wonderful support from my family, I just felt on my own, and wondered would I ever feel better. I realise now operations are so draining, and as you get older recovery may be prolonged.

AUGUST 2005
Needed a hernia operation.

November 2006
Yes there I was again, in hospital following a gallbladder operation for stones. Again a lot of pain and slower recovery.

May 2007
My breathing was becoming difficult and I was admitted to hospital yet again.
They told me my lungs where filling up with fluid, and I spent another month there and following tests was told it was as a result of the previous heart problems, and Drs told me that medication would help but I needed to do breathing exercises to help my heart and lungs get improved circulation.
A nurse gave me a leaflet about Tai Chi and a phone number on which I could contact the person running classes that where linked to the Cardiac Rehabilitation Programme at the hospital.
I now realise that this was to be a turning point in my life and how lucky I was that I followed through the nurse's advice.
However at the time after I researched Tai Chi before contacting Mark Peters I thought *"someone has to be joking!!!"*
The information I found seemed to suggest that it was a martial art! Did the Doctors really believe throwing me across the room would help my breathing!!!
Fortunately I was not deterred (as I was desperate to get help for my failing health) so I picked up the phone and spoke to Mark Peters the Principle Instructor and founder of Kai-Ming Tai Chi Association.
He told me to come along to the afternoon class he holds once a week, specially tailored for Cardiac Patients and have a chat.
 I was too nervous to even discuss what I would be doing as a form of exercise there
My son had to take me. I couldn't drive myself, I was too breathless, walking with the aid of a stick, and felt very weak and unwell. I now know the depression was causing me to feel isolated.

I didn't feel I would be able to do much, but Mark was very encouraging and because I could not stand for long periods, he got me chair and advised me to do as much as I could, and sit down whenever I needed to.

As we got started I realised the exercises where nothing like I had believed, they where gentle and enjoyable without putting too much strain on you.

I started to look around at the other people in the class.

Somewhere sitting, some standing, but all seemed to be enjoying what we were doing.

At the end of the warm up exercises we had a break and a drink of water and the all important chat, everyone was very friendly and I felt it was a very welcoming atmosphere.

Then we started to learn the first part of the Tai Chi form.

It needed a lot of concentration and I felt at times my arms and legs waving about would tie themselves in a knot, but this is what I needed. Time spent not focused on my health problems and what I couldn't do, but working towards what I STILL could do and feeling maybe there was a light at the end of the tunnel.

I attended regularly and as I found my breathing and general well being improving, I no longer needed my son to attend with me.

I could stand for longer and longer periods, until I found I was spent the whole class on my feet!

My anxiety and feeling mentally low improved also along the way, and for the first time in a long time I felt I was in control of my life again.

January 2008

Because I was able to get to grips with the first part of the Tai Chi form, I decided I wanted to learn more of the form than the rehab class taught so after asking Mark if it was OK I and some others started attending the regular once a week evening class as well that he ran, in the hope that it would expand our knowledge of the art.

I found I really enjoyed this class as well, and met another group of people, they where all on different stages of their Tai Chi journey, but we still had a common theme, which was to improve and maintain health, decrease the stress in our lives, and try and keep a good quality of life as we age.

I started watching Marks DVD of the whole Tai Chi form every day and practised not only at class but whenever I had a few spare moments.

It was 3 months before I could do get through the 37 postures on my own, which I was really proud of, Mark explained that the average student needs at least 1 year to be able to do that. Not bad for an "old un" eh.

At this stage I was able to do the form as exercise every day, because I could perform it as slow or fast as I wanted. (The average for our style of Tai Chi is around 7 minutes)

My confidence, health, and outlook on life were so much better.
Tai Chi had done so much for me.

June 2008
Tai Chi in Millennium Square BIRMINGHAM CITY CENTRE.

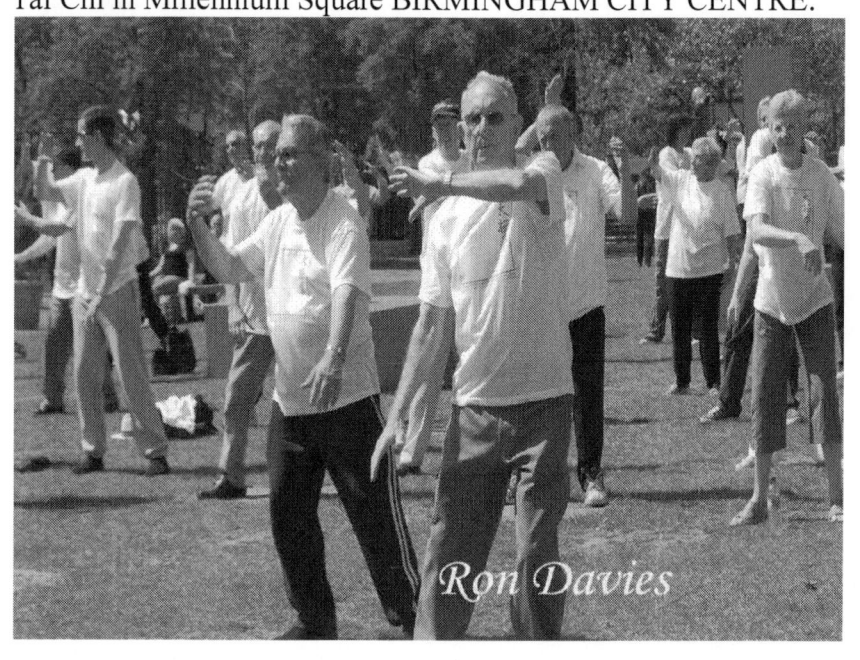

Our Associations members and other clubs from all around the midlands accepted our invitation to come along to a Qi Gong (breathing exercise) display, and we even managed to get 100 members of the general public who were watching to join in with us. Some of the Instructors of Kai Ming demonstrated the Fan Form, and Staff form.

The fans cracking open and closed, plus their colours flashing gave a real sense of excitement and was great to watch.

This inspired me to get the DVD of the fan and practice for a few months, I included it in my daily exercise and if I got a little out of breath, because of Tai Chi I am was able to control it.

I was also enjoying helping in the Cardiac Class on the occasions when Mark was unable to attend and another instructor took over for the day.

October 2008

Saw in the monthly club newsletter a workshop for "Painting the Rainbow" which I discovered when I attended was a new Community project to open up Tai Chi classes in the daytime for people who would normally find it hard to attend a regular evening class or had a chronic medical problem that required that little bit extra attention

Anyone wishing to become an instructor working in this area would be required to attend regular seminars for around a year, at which they would receive information on various medical conditions that they may encounter at their classes, and also develop more structured exercise tailored towards general health, mobility, and well-being.

Mark's wife Jenny, who was a nurse, had discussed with him how the club could move into this area...

When I attended I found it very helpful, and decided I would like to be more involved
In this area

2009

Mark asked me and some of the others in the Cardiac Rehabilitation class if we would like to take part in the making of a DVD for the hospital, funded by The Cardiac Network.

It was a great experience and we all enjoyed it, and the knowledge that it will be given to future patients when leaving hospital after Heart problems has given us all a great boost to our moral.

One of the other Instructors for "Painting the Rainbow" invited me to one of his classes in a residential home and asked if I would be able to stand in for him when he was on holidays.

As I had not CRB check at that time I was unable to, but because I enjoyed it so much and had been to some more Instructors classes I had the check done and in August commenced my OWN class in another Residential home, with Mark's help and encouragement.

If you have read this I believe you will have seen how far I have come since that day in 2007 when with trepidation I made my way to the first class.

The first step is always the hardest, but if I had not made it I would have missed so much.

I have my life back, a new life that includes better health, less anxiety, a feeling of self worth, and many new friends to share it with.

What price can I put on that?

** Read more of Ron's story in the **Tai Chi Journey** section of this book.

Keeping The (Your) Balance

I read a long time ago that research had found everyone over the age of 55 became more prone to falls. The ability to stay in balance degenerated after this age.
Never thought about why really, but probably due to muscle wastage I would presume. (Hence the need to keep up exercise even before retirement)
All downhill after 40 used to be the joke, seems to have moved to the big 50 now.

This led me to ponder will this still hold true in my case, after 20+ years of Tai Chi.
I did find after the first few years I was much more aware of pulling back my centre of gravity when slipping on wet leaves or ice and did have less falls in these circumstances than previously. That was however before I reached the age in question.
So I decided to take more notice when I climbed on chairs (yes I know, should have used the steps) to change the curtains etc.
To take more care on the steps going down to the garden, and really any situation where I was more at risk from "biting the dust".
This focus on not falling over or missing a step, and keeping in balance had a really strange effect. I FELL OVER!
Even practicing the form, on the kicks especially, I felt the need to sink lower into my leg (thought I always did) to feel grounded and hold the posture for longer without having to do a quick kick and move to next posture to prevent "wobble" and feel well balanced.
I had not had problems before, but I suddenly developed them.
It was as if the "balance fairy" had cursed me!
So I thought, be logical about this, why should this happen when in actual fact I am focusing far more than usual on "not falling over".
Then as so often happens you are leafing through a book and I saw this sentence ** *"The mechanisms that create muscular tension and mental tension work in exactly the same way. Tension depends on the existence of two or more forces or tendencies that continually oppose each other. Move, or stay still? Hang on, or let go?"* (this is split in action)

Not rocket science you say, just what we have been told by our teacher from the very first training session, let go of tension in the muscles, sink into them, if you notice tension returning relax more, let go more, enabling you to find your natural root and connection with the ground beneath you, in front of you, behind you and both sides. When you move you move into balance every time. Seek stillness within movement.

I was a Ward Sister on an elderly patient's rehabilitation unit and day hospital and looking back I realise why once they had had one fall my "ladies" seemed to have more.

The fear of repeating their accident and injuring themselves again created massive tension in their wasted muscles, the centre of gravity was difficult to control and leaning forward or more often backward to try and prevent falling was a major problem for the physiotherapists and nurses.

It sometimes took them a long time to regain their confidence and accept that fear created tension and anxiety in the body and this led to being prone to falling again.

In a not to dissimilar way I was creating tension by focusing too much on "keeping" my balance instead of moving naturally as I had been during all my years of Tai Chi practice.

So the secret is don't analyze too much, just **BE** - trust in your Tai Chi practice and principals.

If it's not broken why try and fix it?

** *Sentence taken from A TAI CHI IMAGERY WORKBOOK by MARTIN MELLISH*
article by Jenny Peters

The Quiet Corner

Open Mind (Kai Ming)
The mind is like a parachute - it works best when it is open.

How quickly we make assumptions, jump to conclusions and close our mind. How easily we form and hold fast to our opinions and then close our mind. How fast do we make a judgement, slap on a label and then close our mind.

A closed mind never knows the delight of playing with possibilities, being enlightened by others point of view or enjoying the diversity of human life.

An open and understanding mind never assumes, doesn't jump to conclusions and won't hold fast to any opinion.

Perhaps it is no wonder a closed mind is not a very relaxed mind.

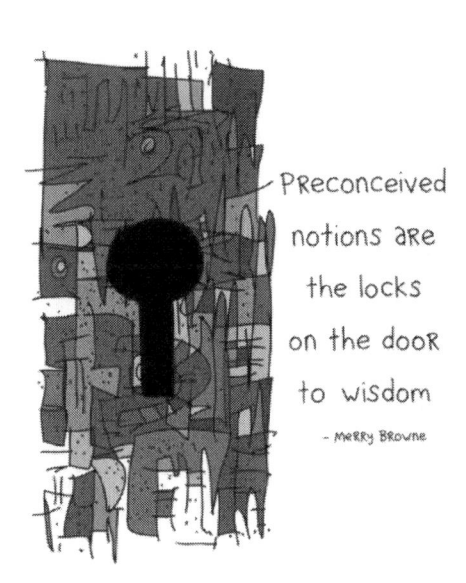

Preconceived notions are the locks on the door to wisdom
- Merry Browne

Banish those aches and pains

When Doctors asked arthritis suffers to do an hour-long tai chi class twice a week, they cut their pain levels by half in just 12 weeks, whereas people spending the same amount of time doing simple stretching exercise only reduced their pain levels by a fifth. Patients with osteoarthritis, rheumatoid arthritis and fibromyalgia felt better and moved more easily after taking twice-weekly classes in Tai Chi. This was reported in Health Magazine in late 2011. "It was incredible," said lead study author Dr. Chenchen Wang, an associate professor of medicine in the rheumatology department at Tufts Medical Centre in Boston. "You could see them change every week. They became very happy. I felt very, very excited to be with them."

It is great that more and more research is being done into tai chi to encourage its acceptance by the medical profession.

Tai-Chi "Soaking It In" !

The basis of this story began in the bath, so I suppose you could class it as 'A WATER BIRTH'.
I was lying in the bath one afternoon feeling warm, and as I thought totally relaxed.
As my mind wandering aimlessly (a common occurrence for me, I like to call it "freewheeling"), I remembered that it is said that if you get into difficulty when swimming, (in the sea) you should try and stay calm and relaxed and you can gain a natural buoyancy and the water will help to support you.
So here I was, my body totally "relaxed", my arms lying limp by my side, but although the water in the bath was deep enough to well cover right up to my shoulders I was not floating!
Now I can accept that my trunk would have had a hard job to float up, but why where my arms still lying there mocking this theory?
I took a slow breath in and exhaled, as I did so I felt my shoulder joints loosen as the muscles enjoyed letting go, then the elbows, and then as if by magic my arm started bobbing in the water, no contact with the bottom of the bath at all, almost like a marker-buoy.
I just hadn't realised that there are many forms of "letting go" of tension and many levels.

Next time you sit in a comfortable armchair maybe reading or watching TV, listening to music try this. Take a deep breath in and exhale and as you do let all the joints go loose. You should feel a gentle sinking further into your seat.
You will be surprised how used we are to "holding on" when supposedly totally relaxed.

Problem is, in its crudest explanation our skeletal system and muscles, tendons etc are programmed to keep us in some kind of vertical position so that we are not just a "blob" of matter on the floor.

Now I may be taking 'coals to Newcastle' talking about relaxation to Tai Chi practitioners, but maybe you could give it a go. (in controlled circumstances of course)!!!

Relax, let go and find your natural buoyancy.

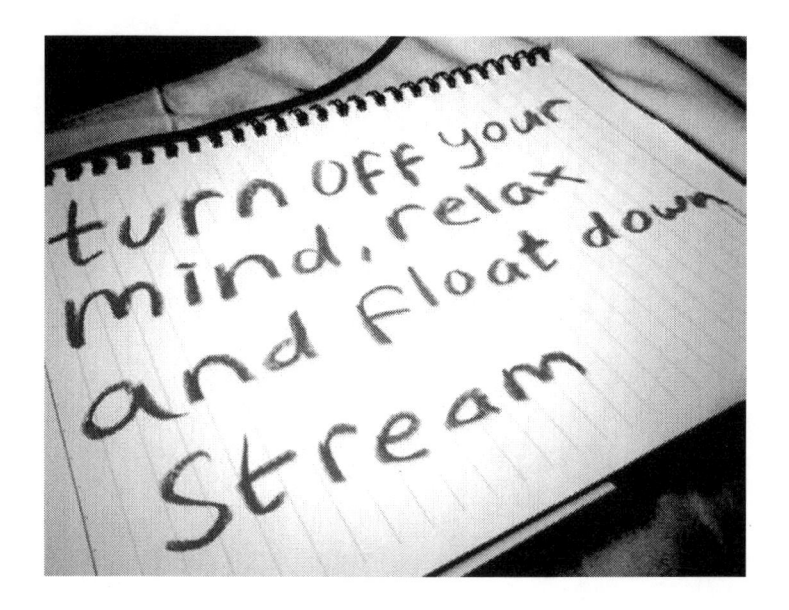

Strange But True - Joint Points

A few things you may not know about bones and joints———

By the time a foetus is four months old, its joints and limbs are in working order and ready to move.

A newborn baby has 350 bones, many of which fuse to form the 206 bones of the adult body.

Cartilage is 65-85 per cent water. (The amount of water in your cartilage generally decreases as you get older.)

When you run, the pressure on your knees can increase to ten times your body weight.

Not a single man-made substance is more resilient, a better shock absorber, or lower in friction than cartilage.

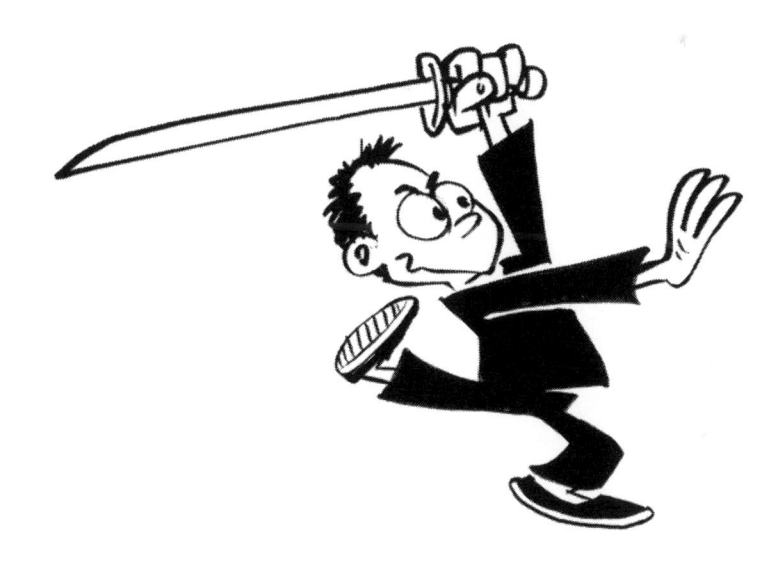

Balance Comes From Many Skills.

We hear a lot about how to keep our heart and lungs healthy, how to have a 'balanced diet' but there is little mention of how to keep our balance system healthy. Your balance system includes all the senses in your body that tell you how you are moving and where you are in space, your brain which filters this information giving it values and structure, and the muscles that act to control your movements.
This complex system needs plenty of regular 'practice':
As children we develop good balance by practising balancing activities - walking along walls, jumping, spinning, skipping and climbing.
As adults we tend not to give our balance system the practice it needs. A sedentary lifestyle, health problems, sensory impairment etc can also weaken this system. Even our multi-sensory stimulated world has an impact with focus more on phones and face-book than the real world around. The result is that our balance becomes potentially poorer.
Luckily you don't have to do handstands to keep your system healthy, you just have to pay attention as balance is both physical and mental, and in fact is an active process not a static thing.

"A man walking is never in balance but always correcting for imbalance."
 - Gregory Bateson

Physical – For some reason I keep remembering maths/physics and calculating 'the centre of mass of an irregular shaped body'. I guess you can't get more irregular than human being! Luckily you can put your abacus away because the process is an experiential one whereby you will learn to calibrate sensory feedback. As balance is an activity (verb) the definition could be 'To keep or put something or someone into a steady position so that is does not falls'; this is where my favourite saying comes into play, "the only thing you have to do in tai chi is to learn not to fall over". Or if you prefer – learn to fall into balance not out of it!

Due to the nature of gravity, the only way for us to move is to falls so a more accurate term for falls prevention would be alignment with gravity. This is where sensory calibrations comes into play – how do you know you are aligning with gravity?

(1) muscles become sufficiently active to facilitate the movement process demanded

(2) structural alignment changes to correct for misalignment. The subtlety of change required is only honed through fine tuning (calibration) which is the true benefit of tai chi practice.

As you hone your tai chi practice you fine-tune your interplay with gravity.

Mental – Quite the mind to be attentive of the present moment as it unfolds. Tai Chi is a mindful practice whether your focus is martial or health; each posture and each part of each posture must be practiced attentively to ensure sensory calibration 'stillness in movement'. There is so much noise in the world today be this attack of another person of the attack of your own extraneous thoughts and actions; stillness and balance is the key. If gravity is the glue that holds the universe together, balance is the key that unlocks its secrets.

Tai Chi a balanced approach – Tai Chi solo forms enable us to hone (calibrate) our balance awareness and this awareness gets its challenge in push-hands where the aim is not to resist but to sense imbalance in ourselves and our partner. Gentle play allows for calibration, active play allows for testing. Push-hands is not about fighting others it's about not fighting yourself, to invest in loss (to eat bitter) and to look to hone further still; this is the wonder of tai chi as your skills can always be sharper…..

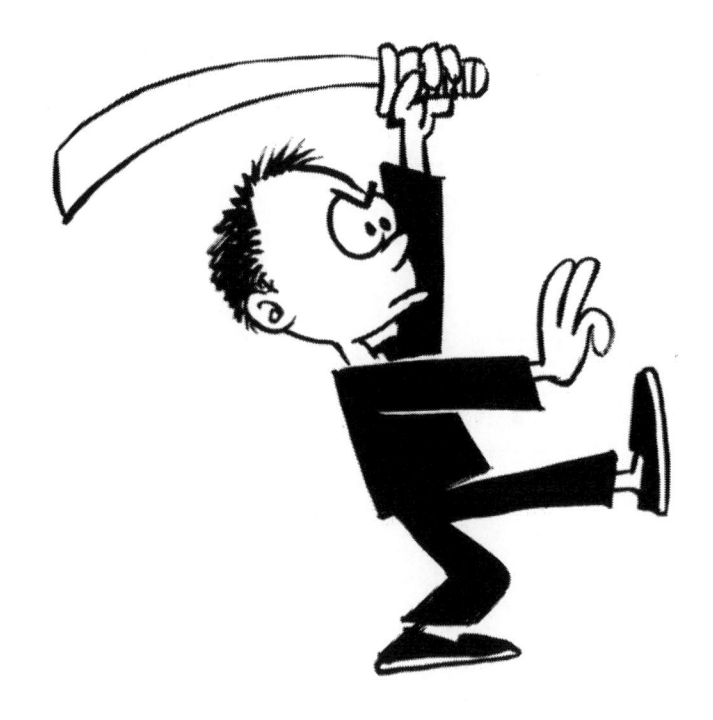

3 Pressure Points to Heal Yourself

By Mao Shing Ni
The next time you have a headache, a stuffy nose, or insomnia, don't fret! Try using your own hands to heal yourself with acupressure.
What is acupressure? Let's start with an explanation of acupuncture, the 5000-year-old Chinese medical system that treats patients by inserting needles in the body at certain energy points to produce healing in the body. Acupressure follows the same principles as acupuncture, but you stimulate the energy points with your fingers instead of needles.
In my Traditional Chinese Medicine practice, I have seen many success stories with acupressure. Here is just one example: Recently, the 8-year-old daughter of one of my patients was suffering from a headache. I simply pressed the Valley of Harmony acupoint between her thumb and index finger, and the headache vanished within five minutes. Acupressure is that simple and accessible.
There are thousands of research articles on acupuncture and acupressure: The overall finding is that these healing techniques encourage self-regulation that leads to health and balance. Research has shown that acupuncture and acupressure exhibit effectiveness in treating a wide variety of conditions, including lower back pain, arthritis, carpal tunnel syndrome, nausea, addiction, insomnia and diabetes – to name just a few.

Ready to try acupressure on yourself? Try these 3 points!

How to Get Started:
Make sure you have found the exact acupoint. They are only about 0.5 mm in diameter, so be as precise as possible. Use your index finger or a ballpoint pen (with the lid on) to press the point. If you are not feeling any sensation, try different spots close to the area until you feel a slight soreness. Keep your pressure moderate, and be patient: You may need to perform acupressure on the same point a few times a day over the course of several days to feel the results.

Acupressure can sometimes be a gradual healing process. For best results, relax and breathe deeply during the acupressure.

Point 1: Sinus Support
For immediate relief of sinus allergies, use your own fingers to stimulate the acupressure point "Welcome Fragrance" (LI-20) on both sides of your nose, where your nose and cheek meet. Apply moderate pressure with both index fingers, one on each side of the nose. Hold for 3 minutes.

Point 2: Relax and Relieve Insomnia
"Gate of Spirit" (H-7) is the number-one point for emotional issues, especially excessive anxiety and worry. Stimulating this point calms the spirit and helps relieve insomnia. With your left hand palm-side up, find this acupoint at the end of your wrist crease, just below your little finger. Apply moderate pressure with your right thumb, holding for 5 minutes. Then repeat on your other hand.

Point 3: Alleviate Headaches and Pain
Commonly used in acupressure, "Valley of Harmony" (LI-4) is often used to bring relief from pain, and is considered good for the immune system. Mildly stimulating this point can strengthen and revitalize you. This point is helpful for cold and flu, cold hands and feet, constipation, eczema, headaches, menstrual disorders, sinus problems, sore throat, ulcers. Valley of Harmony is found in the centre of the web – or the "V" – between your thumb and index finger on both hands. Apply steady pressure with your opposite thumb until you feel a slight soreness, and hold for 2 minutes. Repeat on your other hand.

Do you feel a little more energized? I hope these points serve you well!

The Big B!—— And How To Avoid It.

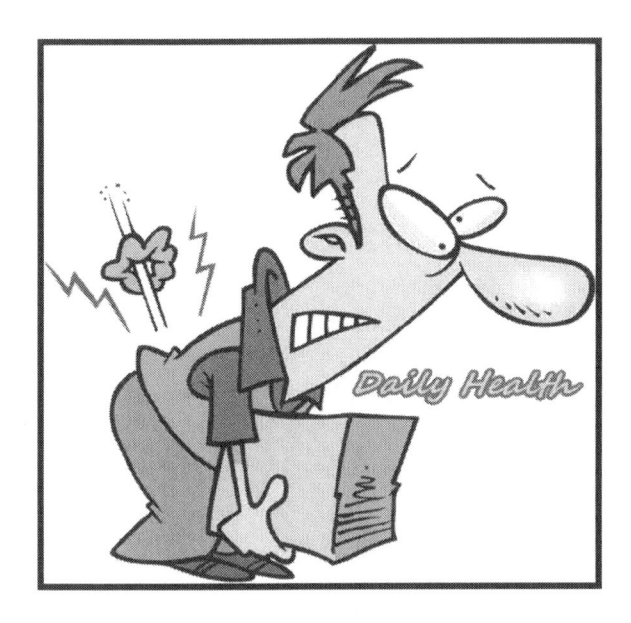

It has been said by THE BRITISH PAIN SOCIETY that 10,000,000 people in the UK are affected by back pain and that it costs the economy £5 billion pounds in lost revenue every year. It may be secondary to another condition so that curing the back pain will not solve the underlying problem, so that the pain can then re-occur maybe over and over again.

Causes of back pain can literally range from inactivity to over activity and everything in between. It is not normally the result of a serious accident or disease, but more likely to result from a sprain, strain, pinched nerve, or perhaps a minor injury.

Many cases will resolve themselves in a few days or within the month; others will need to consult their GP. (Severe or continued pain should never be ignored or self medicated)

Stress tightens muscles that are then vulnerable to injury or strain. This in turn can lead to depression that can bring on poor lifestyle choices such as over-eating (weight gain), smoking etc. that then exacerbates the back pain.

However it is not all "doom and gloom". Awareness of risk factors means that issues can be identified before they become a real problem.

Some Of The More Simple Common Risk Factors Are:
Driving in a hunched position.
Driving for long periods without taking a break.
Overuse of muscles, usually due to sport or repetitive movements (Repetitive Strain Injury RSI)
Being overweight. Extra weight places more pressure on the spine.
Smoking can damage muscle tissue and affect circulation and is often partnered with a sedentary lifestyle (maybe because smoking can cause breathlessness that predisposes to less activity)
Pregnancy. The excess weight of carrying a baby can place additional strain on the spine.
Medication. Long term use of medication is known to weaken bones (especially corticosteroids)
Stress. Causes muscle tension in the back that can lead to pain, depression and poor lifestyle choices.

TIPS AND ADVICE
Avoid sleeping in an awkward position (in a chair) as this can cause neck pain. Sitting in a draught can cause neck ache (muscle ache). Apply heat by using a hot water bottle (protect with a cover so not too warm) now there are also many microwavable heat packs available, some containing Lavender or soothing herbs. These items may reduce pain and spasm of the muscles.

Sleep on a low firm pillow.

Avoid driving until pain resolved.

Stress will contribute to back ache. In addition caffeine, dehydration, lack of sleep and low sodium can increase risk of spasm/cramping.

Treat spasm with heat.

Treat inflammation with ice.

Don't try to vigorously exercise back pain away. Take slow steps to recovery.

Sleep with pillows under legs to elevate them.

Try easy stretches in line with your state of healing.

Postural treatments work in 50-60% of patients
Acupuncture and massage do work for some and are worth investigating making sure you check the practitioner is registered with the governing body of their profession.

Maintain good posture at all times. (Tai Chi and Alexander technique)

Keep moving to keep mobile. Too much rest will allow muscles to weaken and delay recovery.

Walking, swimming, (especially backstroke and using exercise bikes are all excellent ways to strengthen back muscles.

Always bend with your knees and your hips, **NOT** your back.

Never bend and twist at the same time.

Always lift and carry objects close to the body.

In conclusion, simple back pain is something we could all suffer with as we get older, the technical term when you ring for your X-Ray results seems to be "Wear and Tear" and the treatment?——pain killers when required!
However being aware of posture, risks and remedies can make life a lot easier.
Your local chemist is now much better equipped to give you good advice and also they will refer you to your GP· if they feel it necessary.

But guess what? One of the most effective mobilising and strengthen exercises you can do, both for prevention and recover, is **Tai Chi**. It is a whole body musculoskeletal training system. It is also a mind and body approach to wellness so acts to ease stress and anxiety by mindful practice. Just 15 minutes per day can show real benefits with improved circulation, mobility, muscle tone and posture. Even push-hands is designed to improve balance awareness

Have you got the spine for it?

Humans are among a very few animals that move through the world in an upright position. The position puts stresses on the spine not experienced by 4 legged animals. The natural curves in our spine are thus important in providing shock absorption and structural integrity during upright, seated or standing activities.

I remember when I first began training in tai chi and being told a few of the standard tai chi postural adjustments, one of which was "tuck your tailbone under and straighten you back" or words to that effect... but how correct is this? How is our spine designed to function?
Many people are unaware that, as humans, we have three natural spinal curves that are formed in early childhood. We are born with one continuous C-shaped curve. As infants, when we begin to raise our heads, and later, when we push up on our hands to crawl, the concave (or lordotic) curves of the neck (the cervical spine) and low back (the lumbar spine) are formed. The convex curve of the mid-back where the ribs attach (the thoracic spine) is left over from the original C-shaped curve. Please note, some children walk before they crawl and never fully develop the spinal curves. The person with resulting straight spine (referred to as the 'military spine') is prone to neck and back problems as well as headaches related to structural stress.

A healthy lower back depends on good structural alignment, unrestricted range of joint motion, maintenance of the lumber curve, and the support of a sufficiently strong lower-back and abdominal muscles. The practice of good posture while standing and sitting, along with daily exercise to maintain muscle tone and joint movement, will help to reduce the risks of lower back injury.

Tucking the tailbone is contrary to good back health as it can flatten then spines lumber curve, just as over-arching the lower back can put strain on vertebrae and cause tension in the back muscles. In the practice of tai chi form and push-hands the lower back with naturally tilt and release when changing weight and bending your knees. This action acts to mobilise the spine and feed the intervertebral discs which work similar to a sponge.

Releasing the lower-back may be a better description than 'tuck the tailbone' as it aids natural positioning and promotes good spinal health.

The correct spine curves both act as a shock absorber and spring-like compressive power for tai chi application.

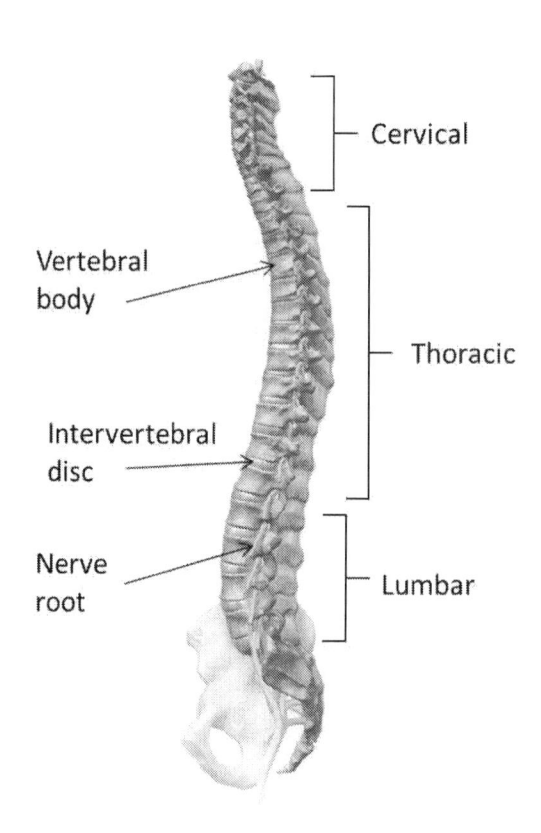

Cervical

Vertebral body

Thoracic

Intervertebral disc

Nerve root

Lumbar

Learn To Walk Before You Run

Maybe you remember the old proverb which points to the importance of taking your time to understand something sufficiently before doing it. Here I'd like to work with this concept both metaphorically and literally by exploring the process of correct walking.

Next time you are out on a busy street, look around you and notice the people walking past going about their daily business. But stop for a moment to really watch; hunched over, shoulders tense, arms stiff and unmoving. The simple act of movement seems a struggle for many because they are not walking correctly.
I admit it sounds ludicrous – starting to walk is a milestone most of us pass shortly after our eighth month of life, usually with the help of our parents plus a little self-taught fine-tuning. As adults, a life spent sitting at a desk, struggling around with heavy bags and wearing unforgiving footwear takes its toll on our posture. Just as we often sit incorrectly, we also walk incorrectly.

The knock-on effect? An epidemic of joint pain – in particular bad backs – affecting millions of us. About eight in ten of us have one of more bouts of lower-back pain at some time in our lives.
One Department of Health survey suggested that 15% of adults are in continuous pain from back problems. Sports Scientist Joanna Hall even developed a program which states 'walking daily will help you shed up to 10lbs in less than a month'. Her method is based on the theory of correct alignment of the fascia, the connective tissue in the body.

I fully agree that by aligning the body properly, posture is corrected and movement becomes fluid while discomfort, such as back pain, can lessen.

The body benefits from correct postural alignment in three ways:
- ☐ **Functionally**: back, knee, hip and neck discomfort are alleviated as joints are correctly aligned.

- **Posturally**: by targeting the fascia, body shape is streamlined and movement more free flowing.
- **Cosmetically**: as movement quality increases, you look more agile, stand taller and look younger.

The accepted guidelines are we should ideally walk 10,000 steps a day but on average we only walk 4,000 steps a day. It takes around 10 minutes to walk 1,500 steps and before you ask, pressing the accelerator pedal doesn't count. Walking shouldn't be rushed as that is what caused the problem in the first place; the pace should be steady with the focus on technique. Please remember it has taken a lifetime of unconscious effort to create the bad habits you have developed, so please start to pay conscious attention to correct this. If you want to give it a nice name, how about 'mindful walking'.

OK, you've guessed it… You know this is leading into tai chi being the solution.

When I first started my tai chi journey as part of the training we used to practice tai chi running, unfortunately my first teacher, John Higginson, missed the market opportunity as some years later Danny Dreyer combined his expertise as a professional runner with tai chi and marketed chi-running followed by chi-walking.

The thread that connects both Joanna's and Danny's approach is the natural application of human design that lies at the core of tai chi:

- Move as if suspended from above – neck long, spine released, hips free.
- Joints free – William Chen said "I don't move my hands, my body moves my hands". Make use of the shoulder girdle (shoulder blade etc.) rather than just the ball-and-socket shoulder joint.
- Connect to the ground – don't "plonk" your feet, sense the ground as you step and release your foot from it as you move forwards as if you're peeling Velcro.
- Connect breath and movement – breath and movement find their natural pace in any situation; tension and stress disrupt this flow.
- Relax (Sung) - enable natural compression to propel you. I missed out on a space-hopper as child so play with the idea now.

Tai Chi is a martial art, a sort of self-defence against life. I don't mind if you use it to defend yourself against an external aggressor or the one that actually causes you harm on a daily basis, the one who attacks you when you are unaware…

Yes you guessed it… it's YOU..!! maybe you'd like to call it self-defence against wear and tear. Rooting isn't sinking into the ground it is connecting to the ground.

I have been asked many times how often I practice tai chi and the answer actually has two parts
(1) the forms and techniques associated with the art
(2) the principles associated with the art.

I practice forms rarely these day but I practice the principles constantly in all areas of my life as to quote Deepak Chopra ***"I am a human being not a human doing"*** and I strive to be present in mindful movement of which walking is an essential part.

I plan to explore the concept of mindful walking a great deal more.

A Black Bag Job -- Sue's Story

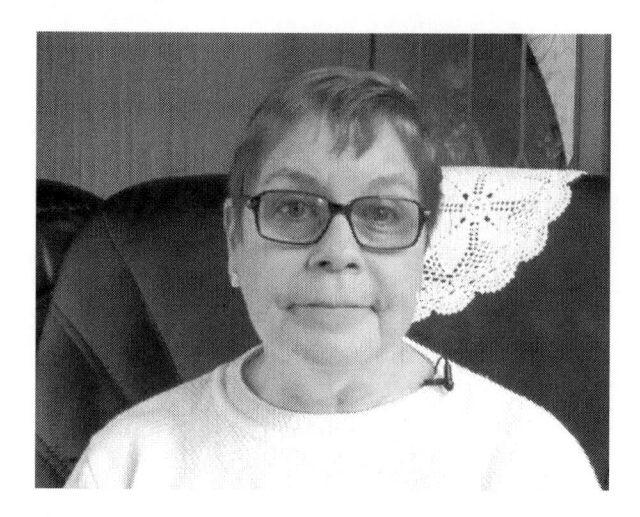

My name is Sue and I wanted to share my story with people to let them know how Tai-Chi has improved my life, and that whatever your health problems are you should never let yourself believe they are insurmountable.
However many small steps it takes to get you on the road to improvement you need to take them.

I suffer with Rheumatoid Arthritis, Asthma, Hypertension, and had a heart valve replaced a few years ago. "Almost a black bag job" I would say to my Doctors, with a smile.

After my heart operation I should have attended the gym for exercise, but my joints where so bad because of the longstanding Rheumatoid condition I wasn't allowed to do that. Despite medication my knees and feet where swollen at times and very painful.

However I did go on the four week Cardiac Rehabilitation course in-house at the hospital I was referred to. On the 3rd week a gentleman came to give a talk on Tai-Chi and it's benefits to our rehab once we were finished at the hospital and moved out to the community to continue the next stage of our recovery in the classes provided by The Kai-Ming Tai Chi Association, in conjunction with the hospital cardiac team. The gentleman was Mark Peters the Principal Instructor and founder member of the club over 20 years ago in Birmingham and the West Midlands.

I, like many of the others on the course, thought that Tai Chi was along the lines of Kung Fu, all kicking and leaping about. We realised when he explained, that although it did begin as an effective martial art in Asia, and is still taught within Kai-Ming this way to the students who wish to study the whole art, many people in the West now practice it for its relaxation and health benefits, as we would be doing.
Relief! I was sure my joints could do with a bit of that!

Mark demonstrated to us some simple exercises to do and also said he could get me doing some of the ones that required standing on one leg! I made a bet with him then and there that no way was this going to happen. I was 51 and have NEVER been able to do anything of that nature in my life. Doctors in the past had tried many different things and lots of tests but nothing seemed to work, because even without my other ailments I HAD NO SENSE OF BALANCE!
Mark smiled and said "We'll see, no promises, but no harm in trying is there? And I love a challenge".

So my Tai Chi journey began, once a week at a lunch time class in a community hall close to the hospital, (although far enough away to make me feel less of a patient still)
For the first two weeks as well as being the first person on the programme with Mark I was the ONLY ONE! So had his full attention. Soon others joined me and we formed a great social as well as rehab group which in itself lifted our spirits.

Within 12 to 15 weeks I lost my bet as much to my surprise I could do some exercises standing on one leg! I also found I didn't have so many falls, because I could adjust my centre of gravity and prevent them without realising why. Such is the subtly of the art.
The group continued to grow and we all enjoyed the social element it gave us as when I commenced going the only time I went out was to the class, and that was by taxi.

After eight months I returned to the hospital to see my Consultant Rheumatologist to asses my knee joints as the previous appointment had indicated that in the near future I would need knee joint replacements. After performing some tests he was pleased to tell me that if I continued on the Tai Chi exercise programme it may be that I wouldn't need the operation for a new joint as the muscles and tendons had strengthened up so much they where aligning the joint correctly and no more deterioration of them had taken place.

I began to get a lot more confident and began using public transport which I had not done in two years. I still had two walking sticks but this meant I could start going out on my own. I was so happy to be more independent, and my partner was more relaxed for me to do this as I had not had a fall since a month after starting Tai Chi.
I was losing weight, my blood pressure was coming down, and after about eleven months my confidence was such I surprised myself and was overjoyed to find I had days when I could walk upstairs the same as everyone else does who takes this simple task for granted.
After a year Tai Chi rehab exercises (and fun) I found I didn't need my walking sticks, which I had been using for 6 years previously to commencing classes.
I felt so good, and looked so much brighter and better in myself that friends I had not seen for a while commented that "you looked a different person"
Mark noticed the change in my outlook to the point that he asked if I would like to go to the hospital class where we had first met, and give the talk to the patients there, that he usually did, to give a firsthand experience; to my surprise I found myself agreeing.

The nurses that ran the class where amazed when I walked in without my sticks, by then I could go up and down stairs EVERY day.

It was seven years since I had been able to do this (one of those in a wheelchair), six years using two sticks and I can even dress standing up. For most these things are taken for granted but I was elated.

It seems very funny now, but the day I crossed my legs whilst sitting in a chair my husband exclaimed "how did you do that?"

Well I had to admit I did it without even thinking! What a long way I had come.

Tai Chi has given me my life back, but it is even better than it was before the rheumatoid arthritis. There are no words to express my gratitude to it and of course to Mark for his perseverance with me and the challenge the 'bet' gave us both.

He and all the friends I made in the weekly sessions gave me back things I thought where gone forever and I will be eternally grateful.

Part 4 – Tai Chi Journeys

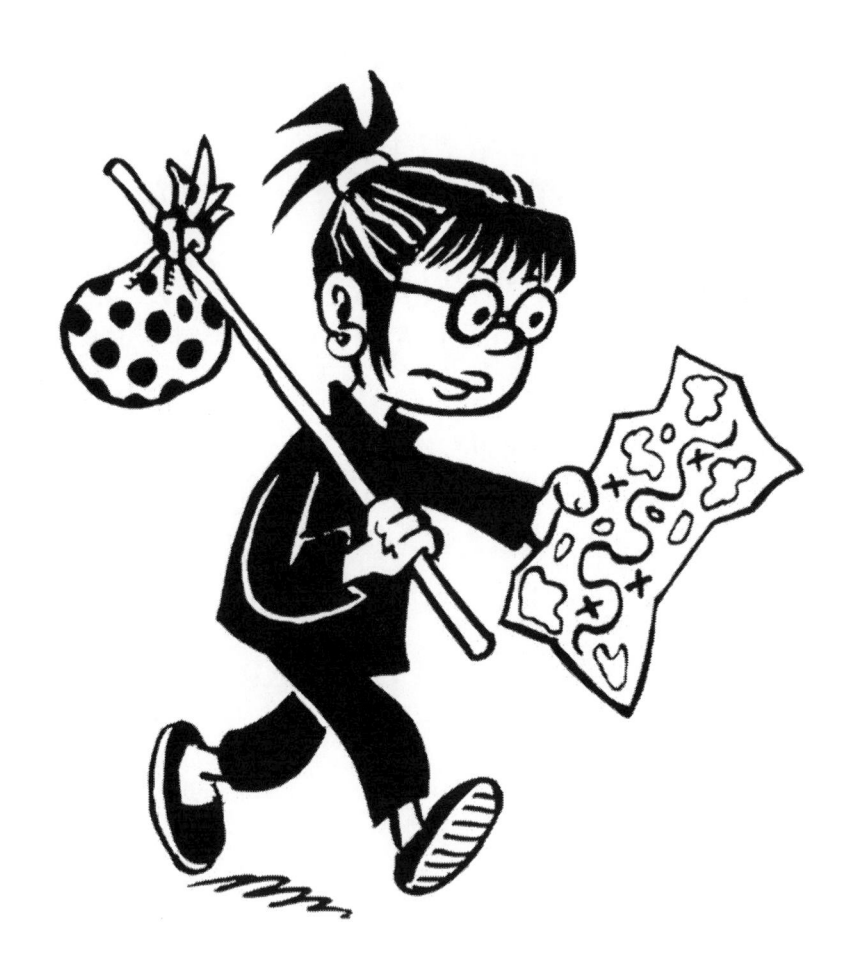

Teaching, Stress and Chinese Martial Arts

Finding a quiet spot on the campsite – it was the long awaited six weeks holiday! -I worked through a sequence of Chi Kung exercises as a warm up before the Tai Chi form I had spent months learning. A fellow camper looked on, and commented at the end, "You must be a teacher too, then?"

Several years before, I had found a book on Tai Chi and read it carefully. I had heard that this form of exercise, reputed to be at least 1000 years old, was an excellent antidote to stress and beneficial to health, and was keen to learn. Unfortunately, no matter how carefully I read the book, I couldn't seem to make sense of this complicated series of postures that all link together to make a seamless, flowing whole.

I have always believed that actively pursuing an outside interest acts as an escape, and as a means of interacting with adults outside the realm of the primary classroom. Part of the stress of the seemingly endless workload is the isolation. You arrive early, sort out the materials for lessons, and then the pupils arrive. Breaks and lunch hours pass by in a blur, most of it spent in your classroom, preparing for the afternoon session. At the end of the day, a quick chat to colleagues, and back to the classroom to the marking and paperwork. At home, most of the evening is spent working, and suddenly you find yourself back in school the next morning, wondering where the last week/ month/term went.

Reading the local paper one Friday evening, there it was at last! A Tai Chi class not too far away, perhaps a chance to make sense of this ancient Chinese art. The instructor made me welcome, and I slowly learnt more about Tai Chi – apparently not just a form of exercise, but a whole approach to life. Learning the movements requires concentration and co-ordination, as well as balance.

Despite the gentle nature of the exercise, I found it improved my level of fitness and was very powerful in combating the stress of teaching. I practised daily and finally I made it to the end of the form, all 37 movements linked into one - well, after a fashion. I suddenly realised I hadn't had a cold for months, and my energy levels were going up, not in the usual decline as the term progressed.

Equally powerful and beneficial to health was Chi Kung – breathing exercises carried out in a standing posture, all joints relaxed. I found a few minutes spent on this each day provided me with reserves of energy previously exhausted by the daily round.

Last December I spent a whole Saturday morning working on the Tai Chi form, with people I now regard as friends, fellow Tai Chi practitioners and instructors. The afternoon was spent demonstrating knowledge of weapons forms, Chi Kung forms and martial applications. "Make sure your opponent is on the floor, incapacitated – but remember, they're going to do it to you next!"
Much to my surprise, at the end of the day I was awarded the grade of Senior Instructor. I still enjoy teaching Tai Chi, seeing the real benefits to both physical and mental health in new students. Tai Chi is not only a form of exercise beneficial to mind and body, it is also a soft martial art. The soft part is being physically relaxed, even while your opponent attacks you. In time, Tai Chi teaches you better balance, leading to better posture, with benefits to joints and muscles. For those interested in martial arts, Tai Chi never meets force with force, using balance and relaxation to defeat your opponent. All these aspects combine, to produce a different mental attitude to difficult situations. If you can relax while being attacked, there's a good chance you'll be able to focus on your teaching skills in the most difficult of situations. One more benefit is better school holidays – holidays you can enjoy more, instead of finally succumbing to that bug going round school.

PASSION - Strong emotion, strong enthusiasm.

These 2 definitions of Passion are taken from the OXFORD DICTIONARY.
Of course there are others but these are the ones related to Mark's closing words of the annual KAI-MING Christmas Party speech.

I quote *"MAKE YOUR NEW YEAR RESOLUTION: TO PRACTICE TAI-CHI WITH PASSION AND COMMITMENT"*.

Unlike other martial arts and sports it is not limited by age or disabilities. It is only limited by your own motivations; if you lose the passion you lose the motivation.
For me personally the word itself immediately evokes emotions.
Like many others if I really want something the drive I put into it soon becomes a 'passion'
We realize students come to Tai-Chi not really knowing much about it and just 'want to have a go'.
We do get the odd one who arrives 'fired up' who has been looking for a class all their life it would seem.
Generally these are the words we dread! Usually it means after a couple of sessions we never see them again!
The reality of the actual 'doing' is just too much.... Tai-Chi is not easy!

This is where **PASSION** comes in, without it your Tai-Chi will be enjoyable but lacking in substance, and that's fine if you are happy with that.
Steak pie is very nice but adding the kidney is where the flavour really kicks in.
Add passion to your Tai-Chi and experience a "banquet"! (Veggie alternatives available)

I feel qualified to speak about the difference it can make because I have LIVED with it ever since Mark began his search for what he believed was 'the real art'

It was not an easy task; there were lots of simple 'steak pies' out there.
He had to remove several 'crusts' to examine their content before he found the one with the 'kidney'
But it was worth it.
He has developed as a person, along with his Tai-Chi.
The 'passion' is consuming once you have it you want it all.
Fortunately for the Association we have over the years acquired students who feel the same way.
They are now instructors, and this year's grading has produced several more of these dedicated individuals.
Hopefully they will encourage others who are considering joining the trainee instructor's programme but are not sure or do not have the confidence, to have a go.
At the very least it will be an extra class and will improve your knowledge of the art, even if you decide not to grade at the end of the years training.
At the very best you will develop *'the passion'* and want to find the essence as Mark did.
Tai-Chi is a never ending journey for him, but a journey he is enjoying so much and which has enriched his life immeasurably.
I find it hard to remember life without it.
I close with a remark from one of our newly graded instructors.
At the Christmas meal on receiving his certificate he told us that it meant more to him than any other scholastic achievement he had received.
It meant we trusted him as a person and his knowledge of the art itself, to allow him to be graded by the club to teach others.
An honour he was overcome with and thanked us for.
It really had nothing to do with us.

He has the **PASSION** and we thank him for wanting to pass it on to others.

Tai Chi Chainsaw

I was holding the logs steady while Bob cut them into six inch lengths with the chainsaw. The logs had to be short to fit into a tiny wood burner, but this put my hands very close to the chainsaw causing some apprehensive tension. I needed to hold tight because the saw would catch the log and snatch it frighteningly fiercely. So... how does a tai chi student deal with tension? *Relax!*
So, I relaxed, held the log with *soft hands, dropped my elbows and my own weight...* and the next cut was cleaner and quicker, with no 'pulling' from the saw. I was still only six inches from a bad movie nightmare of an accident but the effect was so positive and I felt much safer. An interesting lesson.

The next chainsaw job was to cut my own woodpile. Circumstance had it that I was working on my own this time, but I thought I'd learnt the basics of chainsaw handling and with appropriate caution it should be safe. However there was no one to hold the logs steady and no soft ground to cut down into. Two fat tree stumps positioned just so looked more or less good enough to hold a log steady...
Mindfully the lone student took a good stance, slightly wider than usual, and lowered the blade into the log's *centre*. Not quite the same as *push hands,* but even a petrol driven 28 inch chainsaw can give feedback and any unwanted movement in the log could be felt and corrected. In only a couple of hours more than a ton of tree trunks and branches was cut into ten inch lengths (my wood burner is bigger!). Now they needed splitting.

A log maul is like an axe but with a 50% heavier and thicker head so that it opens the cut as a wedge would. *Huang's fourth loosening exercise* teaches us to drop our weight. (This is the 'warm-up' where we bring our hands together in front of the chest, and, 'rolling' the hands down, soften the knees and drop the whole body weight. If you don't know it, or need revision, ask your instructor – it is in the syllabus.) No arm circling with a heavy maul (please!), but dropping the whole body weight whilst standing square to the target, and with a keen eye on the *'centre'*, where I wanted the log to split, it worked *effortlessly*. Six pounds of sharpened wedge on the end of a metre long shaft doesn't need any extra effort to split a log if it is hit square in the right place... until I got to the knotty bits, where the grain is tighter and not straight. 'Mindfulness' turned into 'bloody-minded' and brute force took over but that isn't the point here...

With the yard covered in split logs the working conditions were becoming hazardous, but it is good to keep changing any repetitive activity, so I set to stacking them. Cut and split they are no longer heavy but there is a lot of bending and twisting in picking them up, not to mention avoiding tripping over them. Of course *Snake creeps down* to pick up the logs and turning correctly, without twisting knees, to face the pile squarely for stacking them was the solution to this problem.

After half a day's work I had a very impressive stack of fire wood, a self-satisfied grin and no aches, pains or fatigue. A very useful reminder that Tai Chi principles can, and should, be applied to everything we do.

My Tai Chi Journey

by Leigh Mathers student

"Foorwarrrd...baackwarrrd...ward off riiiight!" The instructors voice was as hypnotic and warm as the Indian Ocean lapping rhythmically against the surrounding beach, as he guided us through the rudiments of what I would come to know as The Form.

This was my first taste of tai chi.
My husband and I were on honeymoon in heavenly Mauritius. The wonderful instructor was quite possibly the most relaxed man I had ever met. He had a wise, serene, "guru" air about him, was stupendously supple (he also taught yoga), possessed a permanent smile, and chanted instructions to us in a very long-vowelled Indian accent.
We were, believe it or not, the only participants in his tai chi class. We occupied a private niche in the hotel gardens, where a heady brew of floral scents suffused the late afternoon air.
I had never experienced such utter contentment.

It was over a year later, in August 2008, when I heard that a new tai chi class had begun local to me, in the somewhat less exotic surroundings of Little Aston Village Hall.
Now admittedly utter contentment had been very easy to achieve in Mauritius, but I did go some way towards replicating the sense of wellbeing during that hour in Little Aston.
People talk a lot these days about going on a journey, be it literal or metaphorical. I embarked on my personal tai chi journey that evening. To the regular soundtrack of soft Chinese percussion music, I began to learn the 37-stage Cheng Man Ching Form – in obviously far more intricate detail than during half an hour in Mauritius among the jasmine flowers.

The standard posture took some getting used to initially: feet shoulder-width apart, knees slightly bent, pelvis tucked under, head lifted as if pulled upright by an invisible string. Some of the exercises involved adopting positions which probably looked extremely silly yet felt entirely comfortable. I was soon balancing wobble-free on one leg while twirling the other ankle for several minutes.

I remember the first time I rubbed my hands together then held my palms an inch apart to feel the flow of energy between them. Oh yes, there was a definite force, as though something tangible and spongy was held here, like a ball of dough. It was an electrifying and lovely feeling.

After the half-hour warm up the group split, with one instructor, Neil, taking us beginners (just two of us that week) aside to start the basics, while his colleague progressed the more advanced members – who had been attending the class since April – further through the Form.

At the end of the class I felt so alive, yet in a different way to when I'm hiking over hills (I'm a keen walker too). These exercises were neither aerobic nor gymnastic; in fact I had barely moved from my spot, but it was all about internal energy. Mine was positively surging around my body.

It took a year to learn the form in full, averaging at one new step per week – steps which glory in such names as Single Whip, Repulse Monkey and Carry Tiger to the Mountain. Once learned, each move is repeated and repeated and refined to the Nth degree, with the focus on different facets. Patience is not so much a virtue as a prerequisite in tai chi. This is an art that can take a lifetime to practise and perfect.

I have well and truly fallen in love with tai chi. The benefits to my health and general wellbeing have been enormous. It can't be a coincidence that I haven't (touch lots of wood) had a day's illness in three years.

I also find I sleep much better on "tai chi nights", and that just 10 minutes of practice a day – a routine I try and adhere to – takes me out of myself and calms me beyond belief. The intricate moves require such intent concentration that all thoughts of everyday stresses are temporarily pushed out of the mind.

I am forever discovering inventive ways to incorporate tai chi into my daily life (a spot of Standing Post while waiting for the kettle to boil). I am more conscious of my posture and balance; I feel physically stronger; I try, as often as I can remember, to "breathe abdominally!"

I would like to say a huge thank you to Neil for being such inspirational instructor! Though I won't be ruling out future excursions to Mauritius to revisit Raj

Neglecting the near in search of the far - Part 1

Would you try and write a book before you knew the whole alphabet, or perform a solo spot with the Royal Ballet, after a few months of "Ballet, tap and acro"? Why then, I'm wondering, do so many students of Tai Chi Chuan feel the need to try and progress in the art, much faster than their capabilities allow? It is generally acknowledged, that it takes approximately one year to actually learn the 37 postures of the Cheng form, and perhaps another 20 (give or take a decade), to become proficient. I have also read in books written by revered masters, that the student should be of a good standard, and have a genuine understanding and ' feel' for the principles of Tai Chi empty hand form, before they would teach them any more advanced patterns or weapons. Here the problem in the Western world arises. How do we the students, judge ourselves both physically, and mentally ready. I myself, after four years training decided to join the straight sword class, thinking I had mastered the intricacies of the normal weekly Tai Chi group. WRONG. As some of the waist movements and focus are reminiscent of the empty hand set, I seemed to pick it up quite quickly. However, I ALSO FORGOT IT AGAIN JUST AS FAST.

At this point many students will ask, "What weapon do we start on next?" This set me thinking, if as Grand Master Cheng Man Ching says in the book There are no Secrets by Wolf Lowenthal, "everything in Tai Chi comes from the FORM', then surely your form should be as good as you can get it, before diverting your attention to other facets of the system. I have been training for 7 years now, and am still unhappy with many of my postures. There can always be improvement, your body is always changing and Tai Chi will adapt itself to this over the years. Each time a Master has visited our club to teach workshops, he has opened up new areas of the form for us to explore and perhaps expand on. Small corrections of seemingly insignifi-cant importance have sometimes changed my whole view of what I should be trying to achieve when I practice.
Why do we seem to neglect the near whilst seeking the far?

Perhaps we lose sight of why we became a student of this art in the first place. What where we looking for? What attracted us in the first place? The most common answers to these questions are "I need some relaxation, I'm so stressed" "I'd like to get fit and, don't want to do aerobics." "My friend suggested I come with them." "I saw it on telly and fancied a go." "I want to learn a martial art that won't damage my joints, and is none aggressive." "Whorf on Star Trek does it, and he calls it Klingon Combat!!!!" (Strange but true). "I like to see my husband occasionally". (That's me). I can honestly say I've never heard anyone answer "because I want to learn all the weapons etc." If they had, I'm sure most clubs would have advised them to think again. When prospective students enquire as to how long it will take to be able to be use Tai Chi as a form of self defence, it is only honest to tell them at least 3 years and sometimes a lot longer, depending on their ability plus their patience, and here we have it, the key word, the essence, the 'Holy Grail' of Tai Chi

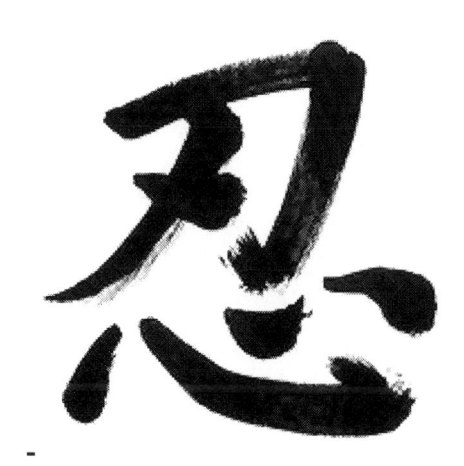

忍

--PATIENCE ---

Traditionally the Chinese calligraphy for this word hangs in every training hall (including mine). The problem is many Westerners want the 'quick fix'. Learn as much as you can, in the shortest time possible. These people are the ones who invariably move from one martial art to another, like a rolling stone gathering a little moss from each (but none of any quality). They want to advance in everything they try too quickly, and therefore find it too hard to grasp and decide it isn't the one for them. With Tai Chi, the more you look into your form, the more you question your postures, the more you ask your instructor, the more you will know yourself, the more benefits you will get. Weapons and advanced empty hand forms are the icing on the cake for the long term practitioner. The form is the cake and the occasional 'Cherries' we bite into, are the sudden breakthroughs that come out of the blue, during a class, when you feel the exhilaration of 'Getting it Right' or understand why you haven't for the last 2 years!!!!

I personally have no aspirations to ex-cel at anything other than the 37 postures; there is all I want from Tai Chi contained therein. That I will probably never move on to more advanced forms is of no consequence to me. The important thing is that I can be patient, and understand, that the elusive butterfly just might alight upon me, if I stop chasing it!

Finally every teacher must take responsibility for the path their student takes. We are all different, our abilities varied, and sometimes we need to be advised and guided when to move forward with confidence or hold back with patience. A good instructor will see your weaknesses and strengths and nurture you accordingly. Who knows, perhaps if you stop and think, the near may be all you really need for now and the far may be a lot closer than you realise! - by Jenny Peters

An instructor's view… Part 2

There has been excellent feedback for Part 1 written by Jenny, but it is a never ending struggle; only recently a student in one of the beginners' classes was walking around disinterested and asked what came next. It seems we are terminally impatient. If the urge to run rather than walk sweeps over you, please read the section below and try a little patience………

Neglecting the near in search of the far applies to everyday life, be it expecting a promotion at work before you have proven your abilities or trying to make a cup of tea before the kettle has boiled. In terms of martial arts it is applied to neglecting basics while striving for the skills of the teacher. Unfortunately you can't put the roof on a house until you have laid the foundations, built the walls, fitted the windows etc. The most over enthusiastic stu-dents are the ones who quit first (generally); in all my years as a tai chi student and instructor, I have been asked numerous times "how long will it take me to be-come an instructor, because that's what I really want to do". Without fail they all brought books, videos and repeatedly asked to move on through the form more quickly, and without fail they all gave up before they finished the first section (17 moves) of the form.

Those who have staid, those who have truly progressed have been the ones with the most patience. I was not really that different; when I started all I wanted to do was learn how to fight with this wonderful art, and all I initially suc-ceeded to do was get knocked about by my then instructor. Luckily for me, I soon learned the importance of building that foundation. Every teacher I have trained with has emphasised the importance of development at your natural pace. In terms of Tai Chi, this is really applying the Tao and following the laws of nature (all things naturally and never forced). Just this week I was asked how I learnt to apply tai chi applications and how many appli-cations did I know. It's hard to explain that I was taught a few and the rest came through regular patient practice.

Professor Cheng is quoted as saying "my tai chi is simplified not simple", and we have all heard the saying "nothing worthwhile comes easy", so why do we constantly seek short cuts. Unfortunately some less honest people use the idea of slow steady advancement and the term 'traditional system' as methods of keeping the £££'s pouring in. Traditional does not mean static; it means to follow a tried and proven formula. If traditional meant static, we would only have one system rather than many, but step back a mo-ment and look at these systems and see they work from a solid foundation. Many freestyle systems have been devised as short cuts, but few rarely survive close scrutiny nor the tests of time; more often than not, they are the spawn of an individual's hard work plus natural ability, once this individual has gone so does the system. Development of the person is often more satisfying to observe, than that of their Martial Skills... Technique is the development of the external, patience is the development of the internal. Focus on the near, on the 'here and now' and before you know it, the far will become the near, and you will have reached the goal the impatient will never achieve. This does not mean I am there, but it does mean I am walking my own path towards it with the guidance of my teacher and the help of my peers.

I'm in Ron's Group

Let me tell you about Charlie, Ron and Clive.
They started at my cardiac rehab tai chi class and improved so much they now run their own group class within our club. Charlie has also trained to be a full Kai Ming instructor and currently runs sessions for age concern following his training for Painting the Rainbow, our rehabilitation branch of the association.

The great thing about these three guys is that they make tai chi fun! As you can see from the t-shirts they are wearing in the photograph. This all started because when Ron leads the group he keeps changing the order of the chi-kung movements and adds in from other sets.... He says it's to keep us on our toes but we all think he just forgets....

Anyway we starting calling it Roni-gong tai chi and Charlie had some t-shirts made.

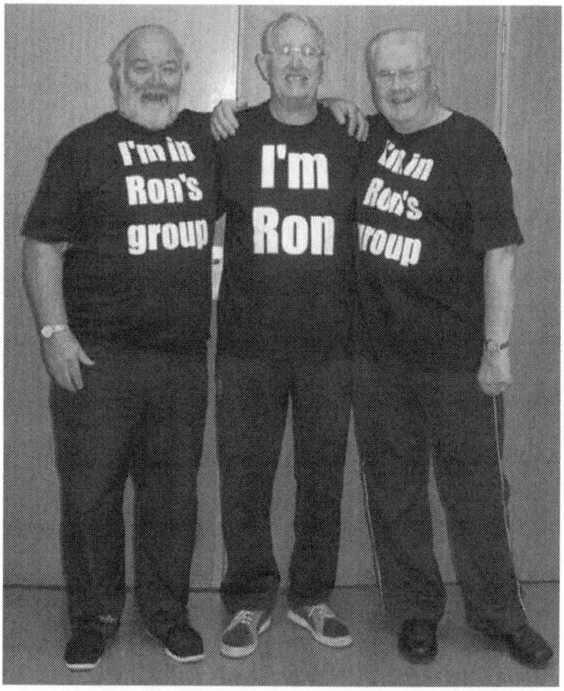
I'm in
Ron's
group
I'm
Ron
Ron's
roup

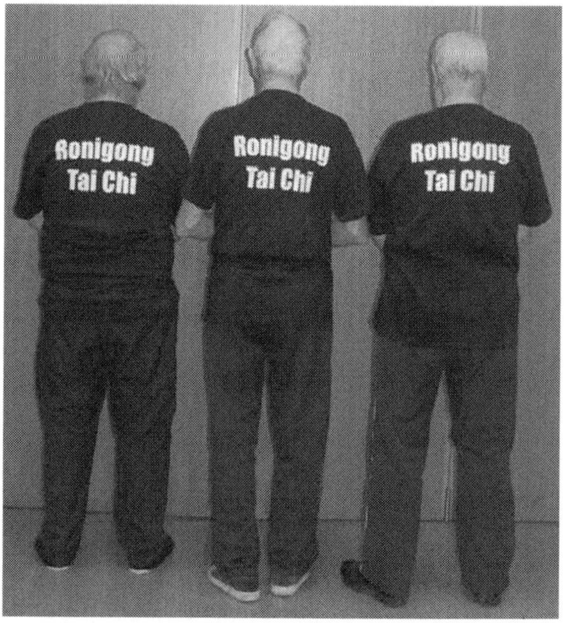
Ronigong
Tai Chi
Ronigong
Tai Chi
Ronigong
Tai Chi

Ron has written an article earlier in this book (health section) about how tai chi helped him recover from his heart condition, COPD and other health problems; in fact he enjoys it so much that he actually taught himself the whole 37 tai chi form, tai chi fan and sword. Some of us struggle just to turn up each week so let's take Ron (who is in his 70's) as a great inspiration. Long live Roni-gong

Mark Peters (Ron's student)

A Students Journey

We all no doubt have our reasons for coming to tai chi, but for me back in the winter of 2006 having been diagnosed with 'global osteo-arthritis' and always being an active person I decide that anything that could possibly help me then I was up for it.

I spotted a tai chi class advert in the local paper so thought I'd give it a try.
I approached tai chi with an open mind and although attending the first few classes on two walking sticks I gradually felt an improvement both mentally and physically. To be fair I was also taking pain killers and anti-inflammatory at the time.

During the weeks that followed the improvements continued; I could raise my right arm for example which was something I couldn't without the aid of regular steroid injections previously. Then slowly, as the weeks rolled by, life came back to my fingers and despite my scepticism I could feel 'energy', like magnets past iron filings, in my hands.

Now 6 years later I still enjoy my one evening per week with my local group. "One evening!" I hear our instructors say. Yes, but for me although I know if I did more I would probably improve more, it's enough for me. I don't wish to reach the level of our instructors (like I don't wish to wear a uniform again) but I'm happy to help pass on the knowledge I've gained to newer members of the class whilst now attempting to grasp the new sword form.

A View From The Front Of The Class

A Tai Chi Journey

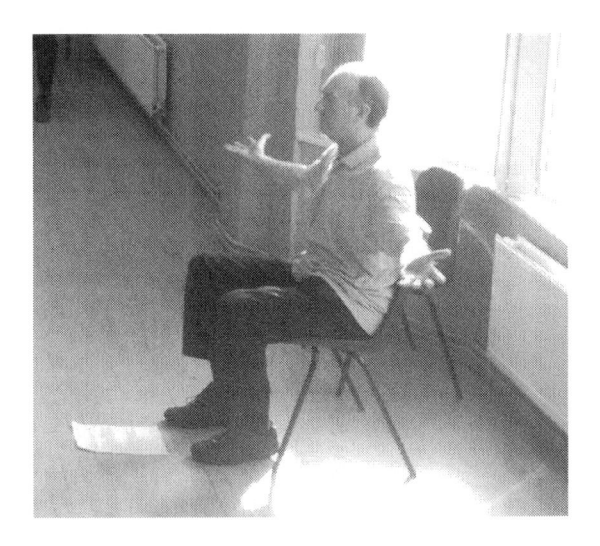

When I first started Tai Chi with Kai Ming over ten years ago, there was no way I thought that one day I would become a full-time Instructor; this is my journey.

My reason for starting Tai Chi was because of the health benefits I knew the 'art' contained. My family health history was rather poor; when I was 11 my father died from an industrial related lung disease (pneumoconiosis) and in my late twenties my mother died from a brain aneurysm. Over the past few years two of my brothers have died from heart disease and one of my sisters survived a heart attack. I, therefore, knew I needed Tai Chi to improve my chance of survival and so far so good.

My first introduction to Tai Chi was from an Instructor who studied the Wu style of Bruce Kumar Frantzis; I trained with him for a couple of years until he returned to his native home, Scotland. I then found it very difficult to find another teacher. At that time, the Internet was in its infancy and there was very little information out there. After a couple of years of searching, I stumbled upon a Kai Ming class which Heather and Dave Jones ran in Lichfield - from my previous experience in Wu style Tai Chi, Shotakan and Goyararu Karate I knew this class was the 'real deal'.

After a couple of years studying with Heather and Dave, they asked me if I would be interested in training to become an Instructor. At first I declined the offer as, at that time, I was working shifts which included weekends and I knew I would not be able to commit time to the extra training. Heather and Dave would not take no for an answer and over the next twelve months coerced and badgered me to relent and so, with encouragement also from John and Lynne (now at Tamworth), in 2004 I and my fellow trainee Mark Walker joined the Sunday morning Instructors class which was led by Principal Instructor Mark Peters. This was certainly a real learning curve as the quality of the instruction was superb with the likes of Don, Ian, Gary and Raj passing on their skills freely and with good grace.

Towards the end of that first year Mark Peters came up with the idea of a Sunday afternoon junior instructor programme which would start in January 2005; the group were some of the first students to take part. This was a really good apprenticeship for me as the sessions taught me how to deal with class problems, structure a lesson, be confident and clear with instructions and, of course, the dreaded homework which made you study and delve deeper into the history and art of Tai Chi.

In December 2005 I was graded as a junior instructor and rejoined the full instructor class. I was now, again, able to soak up from their pool of knowledge, which must have worked, as the following December I became a 'Full Instructor'.

A year later, Mark Peters asked me and a fellow instructor to open a Sutton Coldfield class, which we did. This class is still going strong with many 'hard core' students who are there every week and are always open and friendly to newcomers in the true spirit of Kai Ming.

In the middle of 2009 a crossroads occurred in my life when, due to the credit crunch, the printing company I worked for went into administration and closed. As many printing companies had closed over the past few years I knew it would be very hard to find employment again. What else could I do, perhaps Tai Chi? After discussions and encouragement from my wife, Marlena, and a few months research including advice and encouragement from Mark and Jenny I decided to become a full-time self employed Tai Chi Instructor.

This was a real challenge for me after thirty nine years in the printing trade and was not something I had done before. I was now opening business bank accounts, constructing business plans, marketing myself, dealing with the tax man, organising personal liability insurance and CRB checks for myself, everything was new to me. Attending Business link courses and speaking to other self employed people gave me the confidence to 'go for it'.

Then 'bang'!!!! Six months into my 'new life' another disaster strikes, the company Marlena worked for had a restructure and closed her department - consequently she lost her job. As her salary was our 'buffer' this was another turning point…………..could I carry on as an Instructor and cover our outgoings? Well, with lots of hard work, sacrifices and cutbacks, lots of marketing and pushing for work by me and Marlena, who was now my unpaid, overworked P.A., slowly work started to trickle in. Despite government cutbacks, I am hopeful I can continue doing something I love and bring the benefits of good health to the students I teach.

As any self-employed person will tell you, working for yourself is not easy, there's lots of red tape, dealing with tax, national insurance, insurances and paper work is no fun. Although I will probably never become rich as a Tai Chi instructor, as there is a lot of competition out there, the rewards are you meet lots of interesting friendly people and you can help to improve their health and fitness. Especially rewarding are the 'Painting the Rainbow' classes where people with various disabilities always give 100%, they can be a true inspiration.

If you are just starting your Tai Chi journey you may find that, like me, it may well change your life. It has given me the inner strength to cope with a myriad of life problems and bounce back stronger than before. Sometimes decisions are made for you which you cannot control and you then have to step off one path, make a brave decision, and try a new course. I have left the hot, sweaty, smelly world of print and moved on to a path that feels more aligned to my inner destiny………that being helping people improve their wellbeing which for me, along with the many new friends, both instructors and students, I have made, is rich reward indeed. I hope your Tai Chi journey is equally as good.

Ben Lee's Story

My Tai Chi journey

I am an Instructor within Kai-Ming. I started learning Tai Chi when I was 23. I am now 37. When I first started, Jenny Peters told me I only needed to pay half price for lessons because I looked under 16, if only I had retained those youthful looks!!!
My entire life has been a very strange journey of discovery and it has been mirrored in my Tai Chi.
Tai Chi has been immensely beneficial for me for reasons I will outline below. When I was 28 I was diagnosed with Dyslexia, Dyspraxia, Attention Deficit Hyperactivity Disorder (ADHD) and recently I was diagnosed with Asperger's Syndrome (a type of Autism).

I slipped through the net of the educational system in the UK. No one picked up my difficulties at School or at University even though they were quite apparent In my earlier years I frequently went to my teachers for help but in the best cases they were unable to help me and in the worst cases they made me stand in the corner of the classroom and not participate in lessons.
When I was a baby my parents thought I was deaf because of my lack of interaction with the world and other people around me. They were unable to get any help as there was not even the medical knowledge around at that time of my condition to reach a diagnosis, let alone give them help and advice.
I did not make eye contact with people, because after I made eye contact with the wrong person at University I was set upon by 9 youths. I was also frightened of the down escalators as they were constantly moving. I was always anxious in what I found a challenging situation. I certainly would not have thought I would be able to stand in front of a group of people and teach them Tai Chi as I do now.
My stoop has gone, I have a lot more confidence and My body movement is a lot better.

It is all down to my daily practice of Tai Chi. My shoes are size 8 now; believe it or not they were size 11 for many years due to my poor posture and balance. This is all thanks to Tai Chi.

As far as I know I am the only Qualified Tai Chi teacher and Accountant with my disabilities. Ultimately my journey has taught me that disability only means an inability to do something a certain way, tai chi has taught me new ways.

It has helped me with my studies, It has relaxed me, it has got me through 3 nervous breakdowns, an Employment tribunal and two episodes of depression.

The Beginning

My mum had started attending Mark and Jenny's Tai Chi Class. I was looking for a martial art where a smaller person with good skill levels could defend themselves with confidence whatever the size or strength of the attacker. I wanted to feel safe when I was out and about. I came along and Mark demonstrated the soft power of tai chi (fa-jing) on me and sent me flying backwards.

That was when I started to get hooked. I wanted to learn how to do that. Kai Ming was able to offer me what I was looking for; everyone was warm and welcoming.

Middle

I carried on attending class for about 6 years. I went through all the stages that you go through in your form practice. There was an entire year when Mark had been saying 'Move your waist'. I tried it unsuccessfully and my form was really bad. It then turned out it was your 'Martial arts waist' which is actually your hips. I went through a year under-stepping, then overstepping in my postures, sticking my bum out etc. I have stood in posture for many hours in my tai Chi career. I've been corrected many times by Mark. For some reason you hold a posture and all is well, you think you are doing OK. You look out of the corner of your eye to see where Mark is. He is checking another student.

What seem like hours pass and you continue trying to hold your posture. Your muscles give up slightly and that is the moment he chooses to come and look at you. And it's 'all wrong. Then there is breathing correctly while doing the form. My form has changed so many times over the years as I've pick more things up and my hips loosen sufficiently to do the form more easily. I have also been to every Unstone Grange Tai Chi weekend since it started...

Starting to teach
Mark asked me to help in a class, and throws me in at the deep end. I was one of those people who stood at the back of the class and never considered my Tai Chi anywhere near good enough to stand in front of people and teach them.
I arrived at the venue. There were over 40 people who had turned up. I had been told I was going to walk around helping any new students.
Instead I was called out to the front of the class and stood on a raised platform with all the new students looking at me as I demonstrated the form. It was a very daunting experience.
However It also made me practice my Tai Chi more in the following weeks.

I found that regular Tai Chi practice was beneficial to me. I made Tai Chi part of my daily routine which it still is now. I do the form twice a day and a Chi-Kung set every morning. I was awarded with the 'most dedicated student 'award in 2005 as voted for by all the students and instructors of Kai Ming which was an honour. I also attained my junior instructorship. Since then I have gone on to achieve the status of full instructor and run my own class. It's been an amazing journey and I'm still on it so I hope you're looking forward to the next chapter.

Learning Tai Chi In Unexpected Circumstances
(a Christmas break)

There is a common saying that the two symbols for the Chinese word translated as "crisis" taken individually, mean "danger" and "opportunity", though the second has many interpretations including "chance" and "crucial point" as well as the commonly known one.
At first this seems odd, how can danger or crisis also be an opportunity? I'd like to illustrate. On Christmas Eve 2009 I broke my wrist. I spent the day in casualty and then was sent home with my arm in a cast but still broken and told surgery would reopen after the holiday. It was a pretty wretched Christmas, but at least I was off work anyway and the children were at home to look after me.

Once the break was fixed, I struggled back to work, wondering how on earth I could teach tai chi with one arm in a sling. My students soon sorted that out for me, with good humour and compassion they learned almost entirely footwork for a month and even copied my one armed attempts at "painting the rainbow" and "rowing a boat" when we did qi gong. Thus creating the opportunity for respect, humour and gratitude.

The other thing I noticed at this time was how fragile I felt and I thought about all those who come to class each week with the endless discomfort and pain of conditions like arthritis and back ache. My pain was time limited. I knew my arm would eventually be fixed. This increased my compassion for students with much worse health problems than my own, an opportunity to not wallow in my own misery, plus the belief and determination to make a full recovery.

As the bone began to knit together and my muscles healed from the trauma of the injury, I began to notice, each time I did my daily practice, that I could move the arm a little further and with more ease. This helped me to see the daily improvements we make for ourselves when we do tai chi (you do practice daily, don't you? It really is worth it).

The added bonus was that each time I did the form I was helping myself to heal. This also allowed me to comprehend the notion that energy is never motionless, all things change. Watching the slow but steady healing of my arm and the gradual return of fluidity and motion.

When I returned to the hospital they referred me for physiotherapy, and I was able to compare the exercises they used with tai chi and qi gong. Physiotherapy aims to restore movement and function as close to normal as is possible. I realized that this is exactly what the moves of tai chi do. Each movement of the arm or leg takes a slightly different path to the last, so that in the course of practice each part of the anatomy moves in all possible directions. Later I noticed that other moves in the form and in qi gong mimic movements vital to everyday living, For example, "Dazzling Golden light" (from "Fragrant Buddha" Qi Gong) if you can't lift your hands up to eyelevel, how are you going to wash your hair, or put your jumper on over your head?

Even better, tai chi does not wait until there is damage or wear and tear, but has a preventative function, practice before you get sick and you won't have so much ground to recover.

I learned other useful lessons from my accident, things like patience. My dog (I didn't mention at the beginning that I slipped on an icy pavement walking the dog) taught me a little about using 4oz to move a thousand pounds. After the accident I was afraid to walk her, so bought a "Halti" collar, which fastens the lead under the dog's chin, rather than around the neck, thus removing the opportunity for the dog to use the muscles of its neck and chest to pull.

At first, I still tried to pull the lead as I had done before, meaning that the dog kept getting pulled about and resisted, by walking sideways! After a few days I worked out that the gentlest movement of the lead was enough for the dog to respond. Since then daily walks have become a much more leisurely activity for us both.

I began this piece quoting a little piece of Chinese wisdom and will end with another.
"When the student is ready the teacher will appear". Though I wouldn't recommend breaking an arm as a method of improving your tai chi, it most certainly worked for me!

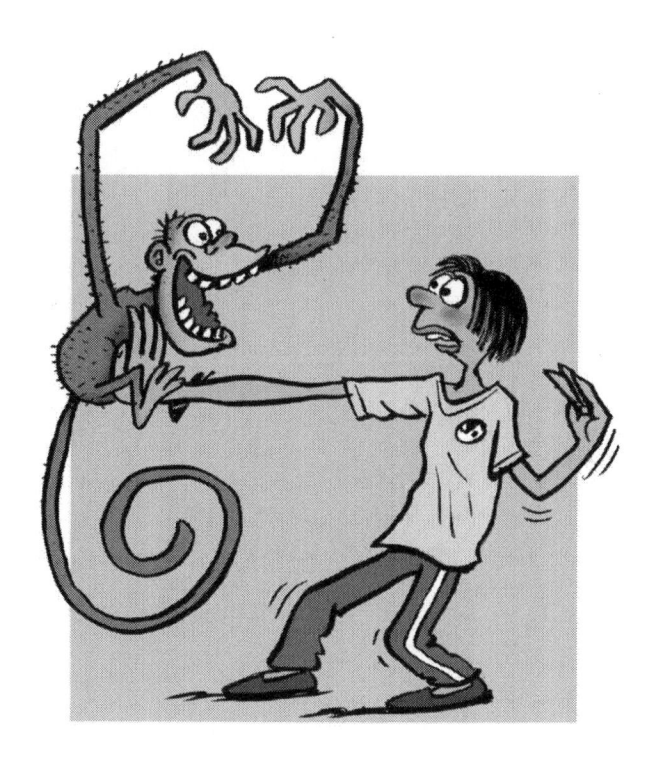

Martial Art Moses?

Almost every day someone phones to enquire about location of our Tai Chi classes or prices, or how long it takes to become proficient, and it never fails to amaze me that probably around 50% know very little about what Tai Chi is, and a few admit they haven't a clue, but could they join anyway!

We have over the years had students from every walk of life and most nationalities and many of them have had one thing in common.

They were searching for "something"

For some it was a belief that Tai Chi could be the answer to reducing their stress, others were hoping it may give them confidence to defend themselves without the aggression of other martial arts, and occasionally both these reasons applied.

Then we come to the (what I refer to as) the "MARTIAL ART MOSES "who will go forth into the wilderness in search of a "Messiah and the tablets of stone"

They will travel miles, spend huge sums of money over the years to train with a prospective "True Master" who has the "Holy Grail" of martial arts.

Become disillusioned many times with them, before coming to the realization that this may not be "THE ONE" and so move on again, in the seemingly endless search for "it" whatever that may be.

A while ago I spoke to a "Moses" who was seeking private lessons with my husband, and it soon became apparent that he would never find what he thought he wanted, because after chatting for a while it was obvious he didn't know himself what he was looking for!

He had had a "need" for many years, he told me, but how to fulfil it had seemed to elude him.

Initially we thought it best to advise that he came to an open class, even though he had tried many Martial Arts before, because sometimes private lessons are not the answer initially.

Observing how you relate to other practitioners and your teacher is essential information in the first inst.

When he attended he spent the entire class "testing" other students (and instructors), and spouting bits of information he had gleaned from his other teachers.

Eventually he asked me if I would push hands with him.
Now I don't indulge in pushing much, and maybe because of this I tend not to use "techniques" (probably because I don't know any!)
I tend to rely entirely on sensitivity, and my partner obviously found this a problem.
Every time he tried to use one of his many acquired locks etc I could feel the hand and arm he was going to attack with winding up, and as soon as he attempted to put pressure on me I redirected it or pushed him over.
He eventually said "you are sensing what I am going to do aren't you? How?
I tried to explain, but the concept of softness and sensitivity seemed to again elude him.
He tried to show me locks, techniques, and meridian pressure points, none of which seemed to work very well.
This rolling stone had gathered very little moss, and talked more martial arts than he could actually demonstrate with any real skill.

He wanted to know how long I had practiced Tai Chi and why I'd chosen this art out of so many
I told him that I had had two main requirements when looking for a martial art to practice.
1. Self Defence, but not a hard external style. I felt that may require the use of physical strength, and also could possibly cause damage to my joints etc.
2. One that would be good for my mind as well as body.

As a nurse I greatly appreciate the fact that we only have one body to last us our lifetime, so we need to respect it in hopes that it will last a good while and give us much less trouble along the way.
As I already had a back problems from years of lifting patients, I knew I could not risk being thrown on to it too much, even if I was trained to use break falls it would only take one badly executed one to cause me injury.
Therefore Aikido which I had looked at earlier was unfortunately out of the equation.
As a martial art whatever I chose, it needed to be just as suitable for me to continue as I grew older.

Tai Chi seemed the answer to my prayers in all the areas I explored and as an added bonus would hopefully strengthen the muscles in my back and around my joints if practised correctly over the years.

This chap was not offered private lessons after the class he attended because although he felt he was ready Mark didn't. He could have carried on training within a class if he chose, but he didn't.
Obviously this Martial Art Moses was still out in the wilderness "big time!"

Then we come to the Moses who for a long period had believed he had found his "tablets of stone". In external styles.
However although he gained confidence in self defence, the levels of anxiety he had suffered from for years where not helped.
He came to Tai Chi after reading about the martial qualities it contained combined with the internalization that would help his stress
For a long time he seemed unable to believe that the initial slow movements and postures of the form would lead to fighting skills even though his anxiety was improving there were times when he was on the brink of leaving the association.
Sometimes Tai Chi can seem too hard to comprehend and impatience can hit us all, but then out of the blue a "breakthrough" will occur and we are back on track.
Patience is certainly a virtue and no more so than in this art.

One day this student decided that all the benefits he had gained from practice outweighed any doubts about the effectiveness of the martial Kung Fu he had had. I think this came about when one day whilst pushing hands he "pushed" his partner so "softly" that the partner hit the wall and slid down with a bemused expression and said **"BLIMEY I NEVER FELT THAT COMING!"**

From that day this Moses never felt the need to return to the mountain and he went from strength to strength with his training. Breakthroughs grow confidence and renewed intent to carry on down the path.

The "Holy Grail and Tablets of Stone" lie within ourselves. That's where you should be looking and when you find them share them with others as you all move forward together.

The Ego-climber

I was having a New Year bookshelf clearout and came across a book I haven't read in a long time - Zen And The Art Of Motorcycle Maintenance. The section below struck a chord following Jenny's article on the Martial Art Moses. Phrases like 'to eat bitter' or 'to be mindful' are common places in martial arts or any field of endeavour for that matter. I hope you enjoy and reflect on what is written below.

He (Phædrus) never reached the mountain. After the third day he gave up, exhausted, and the pilgrimage went on without him. He said he had the physical strength but that physical strength wasn't enough. He had the intellectual motivation but that wasn't enough either. He didn't think he had been arrogant but thought that he was undertaking the pilgrimage to broaden his experience, to gain understanding for himself. He was trying to use the mountain for his own purposes and the pilgrimage too. He regarded himself as the fixed entity, not the pilgrimage or the mountain, and thus wasn't ready for it. He speculated that the other pilgrims, the ones who reached the mountain, probably sensed the holiness of the mountain so intensely that each footstep was an act of devotion, an act of submission to this holiness. The holiness of the mountain infused into their own spirits enabled them to endure far more than anything he, with his greater physical strength, could take.

To the untrained eye ego-climbing and selfless climbing may appear identical. Both kinds of climbers place one foot in front of the other. Both breathe in and out at the same rate. Both stop when tired. Both go forward when rested. But what a difference! The ego-climber is like an instrument that's out of adjustment. He puts his foot down an instant too soon or too late. He's likely to miss a beautiful passage of sunlight through the trees. He goes on when the sloppiness of his step shows he's tired. He rests at odd times. He looks up the trail trying to see what's ahead even when he knows what's ahead because he just looked a second before.

He goes too fast or too slow for the conditions and when he talks his talk is forever about somewhere else, something else. He's here but he's not here. He rejects the here, is unhappy with it, wants to be farther up the trail but when he gets there will be just as unhappy because then it will be "here." What he's looking for, what he wants, is all around him, but he doesn't want that because it is all around him. Every step's an effort, both physically and spiritually, because he imagines his goal to be external and distant.

This seems to me to be the problem of every martial arts Moses out there and maybe even the students who are too hard on themselves because 'they just can't quite get it'. What is 'it' anyway?

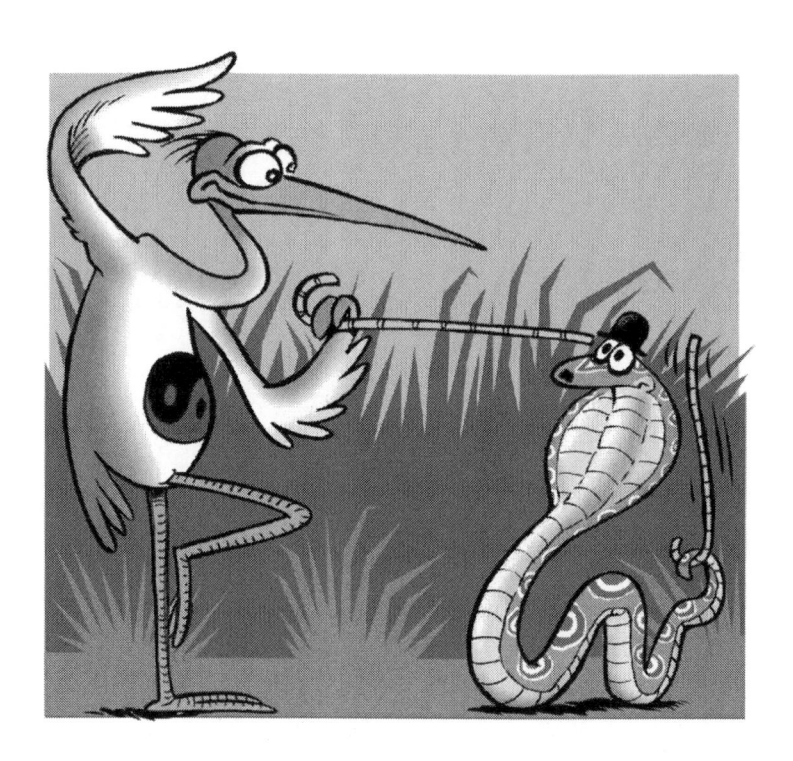

The Tai Chi Instructor (Smooth Operator)

The prose below was written by Jacqui d'Auban as a tribute to her then Instructor Lewis who has since retired after being a great asset to Kai Ming and all the students who have passed through his classes over the years.

He has been on a long journey- Small Heath to the Far East.

It took years, making small steps,
Shifting his weight,
Turning at the waist,
Cloud-hands smoothing the paths of energy,
Driving down depression,
Balancing blood pressure,
Swimming in the air
Away from the machine shop's clatter.

He found his chosen path difficult to learn,
Practising the steps in his mind
Waiting at bus stops,
And like a meditation,
Before he dropped into sleep
Beside a long suffering wife.

He is primed to combat mystery assailants,
Brushing them off, double -push,
Deflect, parry and punch.

Balance is key:
He walks as if on ice,
Testing its power to hold him up.
His centre of gravity has shifted
Down to a chassis slung low and round,
On sturdy Midland legs
Immovably rooted to earth.
He lines up people to make a wall
To push him over

There are lessons to learn.
How will we know when we are doing it right?
When we too can relax our ankles.

My Journey From The Back Of The Class To The Front

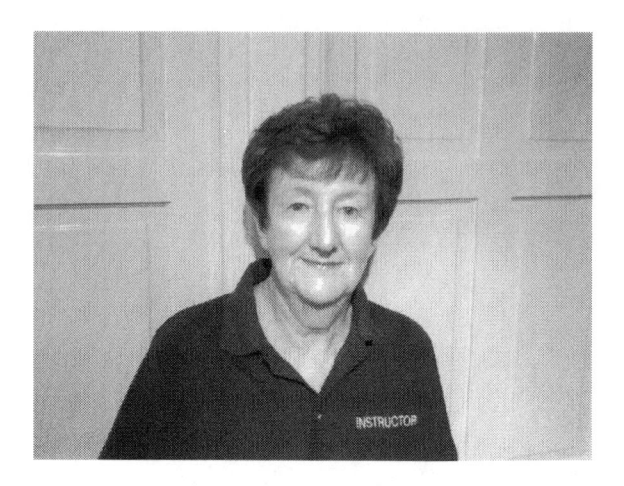

WOW! What a long walk it has been, and a lot of hard work, commitment, frustration, tears and hitting the hard floor so many times over the years, when grading OUCH!

My journey in Tai Chi started way back in the 1990's (when I was in my mid fifties), a bit late you might think to start, but I saw an advert in my local paper offering Tai Chi classes and said this is what I would like to do, I did, and have never looked back (well maybe sometimes!)
For about 2/3 years I trained with a guy called Zak Lee, who was an instructor of Jason Chan, (sorry but this was my introduction to Tai Chi). This class folded after about 3 years and a friend found another class in Tamworth, in Belgrave, which was a Kai Ming class run by a very competent instructor, John Bethel.
Joining this class was like starting all over again, as I had to unlearn the other form and learn the Cheng Man Ching 37 Step Form, (what am I doing I thought) as at times it was very difficult, but I persisted. I do recall though, after asking the instructor why I could not remember some of the moves, being told well at your age it gets more difficult to retain things. Needless to say, I was taken aback, (being polite here) and nearly left the group.

Later on I met Heather and Dave who encouraged me to start training as a Junior Instructor, I resisted at first because I felt I would not be able to achieve it. At the same time though, I had commenced a course to become a Reflexologist and also started extra training with Mark. After a couple of years I made it, I became a Reflexologist and Junior Instructor at the age of 59, oh and also got married to John, so you see ladies it's never too late to start anything. I assisted in classes in Lichfield for a while and eventually qualified as an Instructor to be able to teach my own class, along with my husband John, who also became an Instructor.

Some of the best times have been spent at Unstone Grange Tai Chi weekends, where I have met lots of different characters and done some amazing training with Instructor's invited by Mark.
Imagine, if you can, getting up at 7am on a Saturday or Sunday morning to do Chi Kung in the early morning sunshine, or the drizzle. It was glorious, a great wake-up call. Sunday was always the hardest after our incredible Saturday night parties (John and I occasionally being the DJ's, something John did anyway). Never going to bed until 3am, leaving some of them to carry on until 5am, but we still managed to make it some Sunday mornings.

During the years that have followed, I have become a Grandmother and find that Tai Chi helps tremendously when dealing with children! Returned to college to do more Holistic Therapies.

Because of my interest in Holistic Therapies, I have also trained with Mark and Jenny as a Painting the Rainbow Instructor, which has added to, and expanded my knowledge and I look forward to doing a class.

Although I am at the front of the class these days, it still is an all consuming experience and learning curve, as you constantly meet different people, who expect all sorts of things from Tai Chi. The journey is far from over, there is still more to learn and hopefully many more students to teach. It's been one of the best times of my life, the knowledge I've gained has been invaluable, the friends I have found have made it an incredible journey – long may it continue.

Ward Off Right With A Zimmer Frame

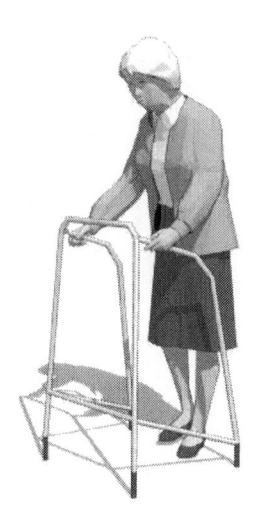

You can't put much weight at all on your left leg, and it's looking increasingly nasty every day. You can only move around between your chair, a commode, your bed and a wheelchair using this special zimmer frame that they've given you with wheels and armrests. You need to get up. You shuffle forward in your chair, bring your feet back so that they are straight below your knees – well the right knee anyway as the left won't bend that much. You reach for the zimmer, which is always next to your chair, and reposition it directly in front of you. You push down on your right foot as if there's a magnet under the floor pulling it down. At the same time, you push your hands down on the arms of your chair until you've risen up enough to be able to concentrate your balance on your right side, get your left arm onto the zimmer armrest quickly followed by your right arm and using the zimmer for support, straighten up.

Then you need to turn. Helped by the zimmer, you have to put some weight on your left leg while you turn your right foot to the right at the heel turning your waist and taking the zimmer round with you until it's facing that way.

You transfer weight to the right, turn your left foot at the heel to face to the right also and you can move forward. It may take a few shuffle movements to do this, but on a good day you can do it in one sweep to the right. Having moved along, making sure that your good leg and your arms on the zimmer are taking most of the weight, you remember to stop and go through the same turning movements with your feet whenever you need to change direction. Then to sit down again, you have to do the process in reverse with a sort of left heel kick once you've got yourself balanced enough to lower yourself down. A lot of the time you manage to remember all this, but luckily your daughter has been to Tai Chi instructor training sessions, and is always prepared to remind you how to lift yourself, as well as showing all the different carers how it works.

I'm very proud of my mum. She was a good student as long as she could remember which her bad leg was. Thanks to the repetition of this routine, she was able to live at home on her own for nearly four months with home care visits, district nurse support and family help. Visitors could let themselves in with a key safe; she could answer the phone, control the telly as long as she didn't pick up her recliner chair control instead, and watch the world go by from her chair. She smiled at us all a lot which was amazing.

So this is how Tai Chi principles all too recently related to my life outside the classroom. We could not have kept mum at home for so long without the help of this methodical way of thinking about movement. Sadly she had to leave her home when the cancer progressed too far, and she passed away six weeks later.

I don't think I could have coped with helping her patiently without the training I've had over the last five years, which I am very grateful for. I now look to it to help me focus on what I'm doing without my mind wandering so much … Now if I could just keep my feet facing the direction I'm going in …

Rainbows End

What The Tai Chi Journey Is All About

Huang Sheng-Shyan felt that Taijiquan (Tai Chi Chuan) was a living teaching, and that it must grow within each person rather than become stagnant and fixed.

He also acknowledged the individual contribution of genuine practitioners of Tai Chi, whatever their level.

He believed all teachers of a Martial Art have their strengths and their weaknesses and that if you trained within other disciplines simultaneously you must be sure you learned from each teacher's strong points and not their weak ones as he had always done over his lifetime.

For twenty years from the age of 14 for he trained with three Taoist sages in the art of Fujian White Crane. Some did argue that this training was a major factor in his later success at Tai Chi and he never denied it, but he always attributed his Ta Chi skill to the late grandmaster Cheng Man-Ching, who he met in Taiwan in 1949.

He kneeled to and was accepted by Prof. Cheng as Cheng was the first Tai Chi exponent who had been able to deal comfortably with Huang's White Crane in a friendly test of skills.

Ben Lo Pang Jang of San Francisco (a famous student of Cheng) told Patrick Kelly that in the early days when Huang first attended Cheng's school he was already able to throw normal people ten metres using his White Crane hands, but the relaxed student of Cheng could escape his push to some extent.

Cheng at first refused to believe that he had not learned Tai Chi somewhere before, but then Huang showed Cheng the secret White Crane training manual handed down by his Taoist teachers, which on the first page had the characters : SUNG, SUNG, SUNG; meaning, Relax ,Relax, Relax. On the second page was: YI, YI, YI, meaning, MIND, MIND, MIND.

Cheng could see that the systems where very similar and that Huang had already achieved the first Ten years of Tai Chi through his training in this art.

Huang stayed with Cheng for ten years until 1959 when at Cheng's suggestion he emigrated to Singapore and later to Malaysia, setting up home in Kuching on the island of Borneo, practicing, teaching, and experimenting, developing his training system and opening new schools as well-trained instructors became available. Later travelling far and wide to many countries happy to share his many skills.

Patrick Kelly, one of his senior students, said Huang was exceptional in his teaching in many ways, one of which was his insistence that it was not a person's race (such as being Chinese) or the family lineage that had any influence on learning Tai Chi, but the person's attitude, practice methods and the help of a good master that led to success.
He also told Patrick that in his experience neither the very rich or the very poor would succeed in learning Tai Chi as they were both too concerned with money.
In his later years when he was comfortably well off, his class charges where low monthly payments for two to three classes a week and if Patrick was short of money he would charge him nothing. Patrick often saw Huang pay the expenses of students who otherwise could not have continued practicing.

In the old Chinese tradition, he [Master Huang] never demonstrated the full extent of his abilities, especially the more internal ones.

When asked why, he said he didn't demonstrate more of them because many people doubted the things he did show, so the chance of many people being able to appreciate his deeper skills was very small.

He did on occasions, in the presence of small numbers of his old students, show some of these things, but on this subject I will for the same reason say no more, Let those who wish to doubt him do so and those with an open mind investigate further.

Like all genuine teachers who teach from their own experience, his teaching sometimes seemed opposite to other accepted methods, but the results always spoke for themselves. In the form, while most teachers stressed the postures themselves, he stressed the changes that occur in moving from one posture to another and, in later years, said the training method of holding postures went against the principle of constant change and could teach bad habits and interfere with the free flow of chi, although holding postures can also produce many good effects and he used it extensively in his younger days.

Taiji tui shou (push hands) was his favourite practice and entertainment. The more subtle and skilful you could be against him, the more he would laugh and return the compliment.
When some people insisted on relying on the external factors of strength and speed, substituting the desire to win for the opportunity to learn, their experience would be a short one and often a painful one.
Throughout the 70 years over which he developed his skills, he constantly sought to refine and internalize them through hours of daily practice and original thought.

Over the last 20 years of his life, I saw the physical movements he used being withdrawn from his legs and arms and then being concentrated and minimized within the centre of his body until at the last, it would appear to all but the most experienced eye that he would yield, neutralize and issue with no visible changes.

This is the stage of pure mind intention (Yi) and all the genuine internal masters have this to some degree.

But at the same time, a more important refinement was taking place un-noticed by most but he attempted to explain it on occasions. It involved REMOVING the intention, or Yi, from the process of issuing energy so that the issuing phase appeared naturally and spontaneously during the sinking and letting go of the mind with the result that it felt both to his mind and the others involved that the receiver of his energy threw themselves.

Such was his humour that once he lined us all up and had us marching on the spot and said that was what all people were doing each day, marching toward their own death.

Then he would pull a few people out and move them farther down the line, explaining that these were people who practiced Tai Chi and that while nobody could stop marching toward their death, they could move a little farther back down the queue!!!

Information taken from the writings of Patrick Kelly Senior student and devotee of Huang Sheng-Shyan

Part 5 – Form & Function

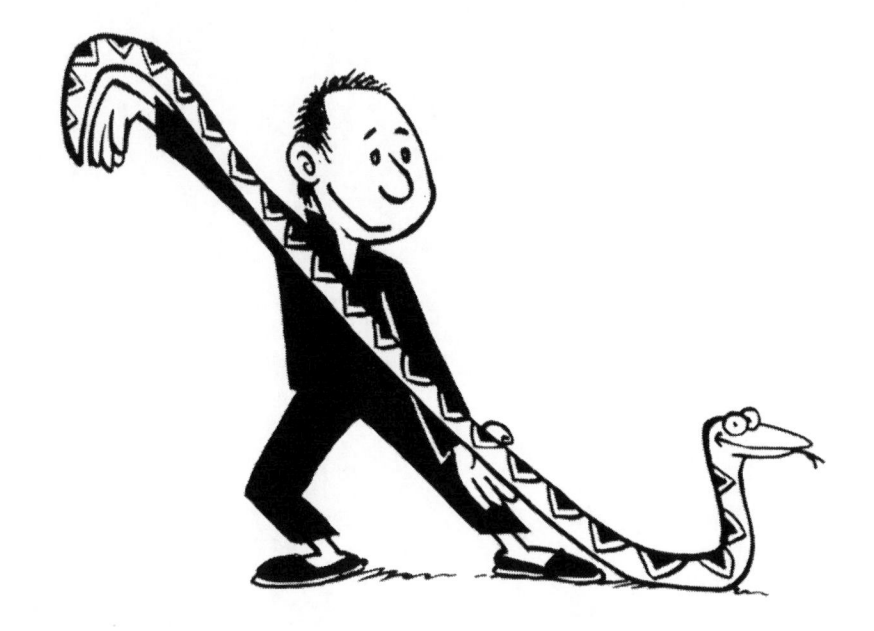

KAI MING (Open Minded)

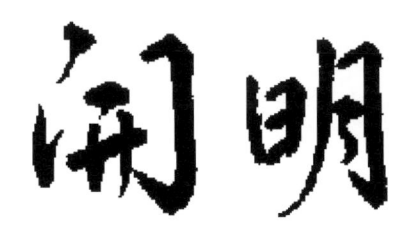

闲 明

OPEN   MINDED

When Mark was looking for inspiration for a name for our organization he decided to research, along with others in the club at the time, (who could read Mandarin or Cantonese) the language and etiquette of the Chinese culture, as it was very important that we found a name that conveyed what we hoped we stood for.
We found because of this how important it was to have the correct characters used together properly.
It was a great learning curve but it was well worth the effort to express our feelings as a group of people joined under one banner to promote all Tai Chi that has the true spirit of the art, and share the way of "The Good Heart"
I read the following in an old magazine from the USA and I believe they had taken it from a book produced in Malaysia. I noticed how relevant this extract was to the name of our Association.

"Taijiquan is not a martial art meant for bragging or antagonistic purposes.
A Taijiquan exponent needs to understand the principles and philosophy of it.
No one should deviate from these principles and this philosophy.
The movements can be developed and modified but the principles are eternal.
The external forms may differ from person to person, but the principles are standard and unvarying.
Because of this, there is no basis for differentiation by schools.

Instead, a spirit of a single family should prevail.
Common interest in the art should take precedence over personal interest.
An open attitude should emerge, bearing in mind the intention of the founder and our predecessors to propagate the philosophy of Taijiquan throughout the world so as to improve the health of mankind physically and mentally."

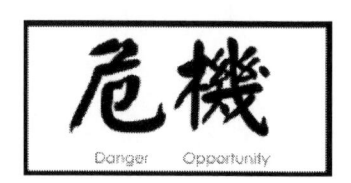

危機
Danger   Opportunity

When written in Chinese, the word 'crisis' (Wei Gee) is composed of two characters. One represents danger and the other represents opportunity.
JOHN F. KENNEDY

Alice In Wonderland And Tai Chi!

There are many paths that lead to enlightenment and sometimes we are led to them in strange ways.
One day I was clearing out my bookcase in readiness to move it to another room.
Amongst the books I have collected over the years are many children's classics.
They are a mixed bag of Enid Blyton famous five adventure stories, right up to favourites from my daughter's childhood like Paula Danzingr's "The Cat Ate My Gymslip"!
I was barley noticing what was there, as over the years they have become just part of the scenery awaiting the arrival of grandchildren to relive the magic of the stories contained within the ageing pages.

Suddenly my eyes were drawn to the title of a little blue book
"ALICE IN WONDERLAND"
Strangely I cannot remember if I ever read the actual book or indeed if it was ever read to me, but I do remember having surreal dreams that where quite frightening at the time, that involved some of the situations and characters Alice became involved in during the story.
We all know or have heard of this classic "children's story" by Lewis Carroll but thinking back to when I had bought it originally it was with the intention of reading it as an adult.

This may sound a strange thing to do, but as I have said sometimes our actions are guided for a reason. Never ignore an instinctive action.

With this in mind over the last few days I have snatched some time to do just this and my gut feelings have now justified themselves.
The edition I have has the reproduction of the original illustrations and I realised how nightmarish some of them where, but the actual story is lovely and the characters absurd, funny, and magically surreal all at once.

Now we come to the point of this article (is that a sigh of relief I hear)

Have you ever heard of the CAUCUS-RACE?

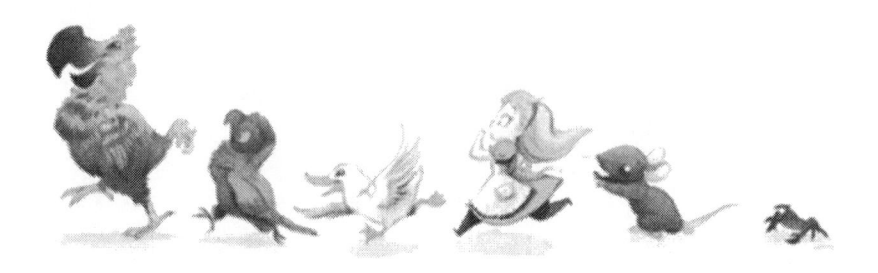

One chapter in the book is about Alice's adventures when she has been reduced in size.
She and a mixture of birds and animals fall accidentally into one of her tears that she cried when she had been a 9ft giant, so as you can imagine it is like a sea and they all swim for their lives!
When they eventually get on dry land the creatures discuss how they can get dry quickly.
The Dodo who seems to be the wisest amongst them suggests A CAUCUS-RACE!
Even Alice had no idea what this was, so the Dodo began to explain and demonstrate thus——

First he marked out a race –course, in a sort of circle, (doesn't have to be exact)
Then all the wet participants were placed here and there around the course.
There was no 1 2 3 go! They could begin running when they liked, and stop when they liked, so that it was not easy to know when the race was over.
However, when they had been going round for about ½ an hour and seemed dry again, the Dodo suddenly called out "The race is over!"
They crowded round all eager to know who had won, in the hope of receiving a prize and admiration.
The Dodo thought long and hard before he announced diplomatically "Everybody has won!" and all must have prizes.

It seemed to me when I read this, that it correlated very well with how we practice Tai Chi.

We all start at different points in our life along the Tai Chi path, and so other students in the class may be ahead of us in their knowledge of the art, but like the Caucus-Race there is no need to compete really, it is our own Ego's that want the prize, ethos, praise, attention whatever you choose to call it

Really also like the race we are ALL WINNER'S!

The prize for us is the satisfaction of practice, when we feel our form is getting better, when we feel the focus is improving, when we feel the stress of everyday life lift as we leave the session with our fellow students.

That DODO was a wise old bird (however not wise enough to avoid extinction! But maybe as with many things MAN helped in his demise.)

The Bubbling Well.

Use it or lose it!

There are many principles to follow when practising your Tai Chi.
Relax, focus on the Dan-tian, move as a unit, keep the spine straight, sink the hips, keep knees slightly bent, etc
Most teachers teach these essentials, and they can be found in the classics if you want to refine certain aspects for yourself and enjoy research.
Something that is agreed upon as being important is the spot behind the ball of the foot that we sink into when doing the form; it is known as the "Bubbling Well" (Yongquan)...
It is believed that this is where the energy flows through our bodies and allows us to connect with the earth.
Professor Cheng Man-Ch'ing called the Bubbling Well, the point at the top of your head (Ba Hui), and the Dan-tian the 3 treasures of Tai Chi.
We develop our "Root" (good stability) from relaxing and sinking into the spot known as this Well.
A connected root is the key to not being pushed. Anyone who enjoys push hands and practices regularly understands the importance of developing their focus on this area.
The foot contains 52 of the 66 bones of the lower appendicular skeleton.
The Chinese believe it is the beginning or ending point of 6 of the 12 major meridians.
This is why foot reflexology and massage can be so effective.
The foot bones form something unique to their area of the body, the arches.

There are 3 of these on each foot that support the whole body weight and therefore our foundation.
They are the medial longitudinal arch, the lateral longitudinal arch, and the transverse arch.
These 3 arches have three points that touch the ground, so form a tripod for stability and shock absorption.

In terms of bio-mechanics of our body, our centre of gravity is the Dan-tian, and it is balanced over the arches of our feet.

Therefore to push an opponent's centre of gravity will take away the stability formed by theses arches, and in turn break there root. Whether you are interested in push hands or not it is still helpful to focus on this point during your Tai Chi practise as it will improve body alignment and overall stability.

On Teachers And Training

Lao Tzu once described three orders of teachers
The lowest is feared and respected.
The second is loved and admired
And the highest teachers without being perceived as a teacher at all; he or she is only a Friend.
Which I guess gives weight to the statement "A true Master goes unnoticed"

The next paragraph is taken from an article in TAI CHI magazine published in America in 1982 but I feel is ageless wisdom. It was written by a teacher from the East Coast who wished to remain anonymous. To perfect our Tai Chi with a concomitant increase in our ego will not work. We will end up merely as skilled technicians.
To such a one the old Taoist saying applies, ***"When the wrong man uses the right means The right means work in the wrong way!"***

Why seek for Gurus? Search instead for a WAY. When you find it, open yourself to it. Guru's have enough problems without you. For to be a Guru is to dominate, and to dominate is to forfeit freedom. A Guru can only introduce you to a way You must take it. Or better yet, let it take YOU!

Important Points

Many times I say in class *"You only have only one really important thing to do in Taiji, and that is to not fall over..."*

What I mean by this is you should learn to **'fall through'** your body and connect to the earth, not fall over your body or float with no real connection to the earth. Uprooting is simply removing your connection to the ground and projecting you in a chosen direct. Because few pay attention to their connection, it is a very simple 'effortless' process to uproot them. Taiji practice is to relax, not resist, and develop a natural connection and natural balance; form postures are a means of testing and developing this relaxation. Relaxed muscles will naturally support the load rather than just hold it up
through muscular tension. If you find standing post exercises too difficult then try them seated; they are not just to develop leg strength but relaxed muscular awareness....

Try an awareness exercises - this can be done with a partner or a reasonably weighted object - you aim is to effortlessly move this item.
- (1) make relaxed contact and close your eyes
- (2) FEEL the weight or resistance of this item fall though you and connect to the ground, do not resist
- (3) try to relax between this item and the ground, feeling all tensions and resistance let go until your whole body falls naturally into place to effortlessly support this item.
- (4) now release to move or lift this item.... If you have it right then it will move with seemingly no real effort on your part; if not just relax and try again.....

Once you feel this free power you will never want to strain again and you are on a wondrous journey.

Training tips

Many think of *double-weightedness* as having your weight in both legs rather than being 'single-weighted' with the majority of your weight in one leg, creating a sound axis. Well this is true, but not the whole picture. We need overcome double weighted in the mind as well. An easy example of this would be having a conversation with somebody where you are both talking regardless of what the other is saying i.e. both having your own mind/conversation; you must have experienced this at some time…
Another example would be in martial practice when we decide the application we will use regardless of the attach applied; generally we fudge it with a little brute force and good luck. Listening is an essential skill in life and as we practice a life art, why should it be any different. 'Giving up to follow others' is a good example of listening as is my old favourite, "Shut up, I'm talking". Well, OK, I am the instructor…

How many times do you try to push with no output except losing balance yourself; maybe try again and listen to the other person first. Build an interaction, blend with your partner, take part in the interaction and DO NOT impose yourself in any way on the other party. Train to be single-weighted, open, adaptable and balanced (both physically and mentally). Learn to understand what and who we are.

I realise this can sound a little heavy, but no need for it to be. Make it fun; by playing games of interaction on class you'll find it filters into your everyday life; maybe you'll even become a better conversationalist.

Subtle skills of tai chi

I am frequently asked about the subtle skills of Taiji and the use of strength etc., so I have chose to briefly outline the 5 main energies.
1. Adhering/sticking
2. Listening
3. Interpreting
4. Neutralizing
5. Issuing

1. Sticking or Adhering.
This is the first energy and involves sticking to and blending with your partner or attacker. This allows you to follow the force without affecting it, to stay light and sensitive, making it difficult for the other person to advance or retreat without you being there. Think of catching a cricket ball, off reaching out to it and following it back with it lightly held in your hands.

2. Listening
Now you have stuck to your partner, you have to listen through your newly developed sensitive touch. Relaxation allows us to be more sensitively to touch, the environment around us and the actions of the other person. How often have you tried to have a conversation with another person who does not listen only talks; they are generally unaware and insensitive to your input. This is the same (and more so) to the skill of listening through touch. IF WE CAN NOT FEEL THEM THEN WE ARE DEAF AND BLIND TO THEM.

3. Interpreting
How can we interpret without listening? How can we be sensitive to and decipher our partners intentions without our listening skills? Now we can listen we can interpret; are they advancing, retreating, off-balance, overextending. We can interpret their intentions and know their centre. Everything appears to slow down and you have time to respond rather than react blindly; you KNOW what is expected to happen and can now deal with it.

4. Neutralizing

This is like catching the cricket ball and feeling its direction; this allows you to catch it smoothly and neutralise its force. If you have connected with, listen to and understood an incoming intention then neutralising it is only a natural response. This subtle adjustment allows you to gain the advantaged position and put the opponent off-balance both mentally and physically. Wherever they move, whatever they do will only serve to disadvantage them more...

5. Issuing

Ahhh... At last I hear you say (OK I said it). Too many rush too quickly to this one... Without the previous four occurring correctly, issuing is more likely to be brute force than effortless power (intrinsic power). No tension can be allowed to manifest itself, all should remain relaxed and the issue should feel like an unresistable energy. This energy can feel like being swept along on a great wave or short and sharp like an electric shock, both have their uses but neither have any tension.

Many books describe these in greater detail; I hope this brief outline helps. Above all notice there is an order to learn and use them in. Do not jump stages or rush ahead to quickly. You may have some success but this can just as easily be down to unskilled partners than to your own development. Never be fooled into thinking you are better than you are, look what happened to the gunslingers of the old West... Practice diligently and the skills will develop naturally...

Balance And Coordination

Tai Chi is a sophisticated form of whole body Neuromuscular-skeletal movement re-education.
With good use, the body moves easily - with balance and coordination.

We frequently and unconsciously hold excessive tension in our musculature, especially in our large peripheral muscles. Without the experience of ease that can be provided by a qualified teacher, we think of this tension as normal. The physical and mental stresses and strains of everyday life (and our individual reactions towards these) result in tension throughout our bodies. This tension interferes with efficient muscular recruitment patterns, and can lead to the establishment of a series of inefficient movement patterns: the habitual recruitment of excessive muscular tension to carry out daily activities such as walking, running, household tasks or performing a mobilization technique.

In Tai Chi we do not want students to strengthen, stretch or hold specific muscles to achieve a desired anatomical posture. Instead students are guided into seeing and feeling how little muscular effort is really required to dynamically balance their skeletons (learn to do less). Often these new movement patterns initially feel unfamiliar, because the new patterns allow us to move with more ease and grace. It can come as a complete surprise that we are able to move and use our bodies more effectively, without resorting to our habitual muscular tension patterns.

Tai Chi is all about letting go; about not doing and just 'being'. Initially this appears difficult but remember you have taken most of your life to build habits that you currently believe to be natural movement and balance; it will take a few lessons to fix....

Look at the first movement, preparations (Yu bei shi). It is more than just getting to shoulder width; it is about become aware of where you are in relationship to the ground and where your feet are in relationship to the rest of you. What is shoulder width? Did you turn your waist to turn your foot or just turn your foot? Most of us do not pay attention below waist height as it is outside of our field of vision, but if we do not connect to the ground effectively we are setting up tensions from the off...

The medical profession even have a name for it, "proprioceptive feedback"; this simply means a sense of muscular activity and joint positioning.

Take your time with the movements and pause before the next posture; give yourself chance to feel the feedback, feel your feet under your and release your weight into the ground. DO NOT move on until you can feel free and balanced.
Kinaesthetic awareness or the ability to know where your body parts are in 3-dimensional space, is also trained and is required for every movement we make.

Once we know how and where we are, we can freely balance and relax. From this we develop agility. Agility is what allows us to move gracefully, wasting little motion. From this understanding we can become effortlessly effective; we can choose to respond effectively to every situation freely and fluidly without force or interruptions...

The Form
by Mark Carter - Tamworth Student

We stand poised and begin to think
Thumbs at our thigh sides As we begin to sink
Our elbows go wide as we begin to flow
The answer here is to take it slow.

Turn to the right and then to the other way
Feet shoulders width we begin to sway
Up and down are arms out wide
Protecting ourselves from the front and side

Breathe in and out and regulate
The slower the better makes you feel great
Ward off left and then to the right
Roll back, push hands, make them take flight

Remember to root yourself to the ground
Adopt single whip as you go round
Hands high and shoulder strike
Step back white crane in flight

Brush knee to the left and play guitar
Brush knee to the left well done so far
Close up parry, punch and push double
Cross hands, tiger to the mountain your opponents in trouble

Roll back and push with single whip
We've done this before I hear you quip
Fist under elbow, monkey's to feed
Step back, pull down to stop their greed

Round we go cloud hands a must
Step out, step in it's the slowness we lust
Step out wide and get your feet right
Step up, to golden cock, a kick is in sight

Three kicks in all at this vital stage
Brush left and right a low blow I'll wage
Roll back double push single whip once more
Four corners now to even the score

Ward off left, again to the right
The end of the form is now in sight
Snake creeps down, to seven stars
Ride the tiger feel the scars

Once around and touch the heel
Bend that bow prepare to peel
Off to the left to hide your punch
Apparent closing is my hunch

As we bring it to a close
We strike a proud and standing pose
Hands back to the side we've done it right
All that's left is to say good night

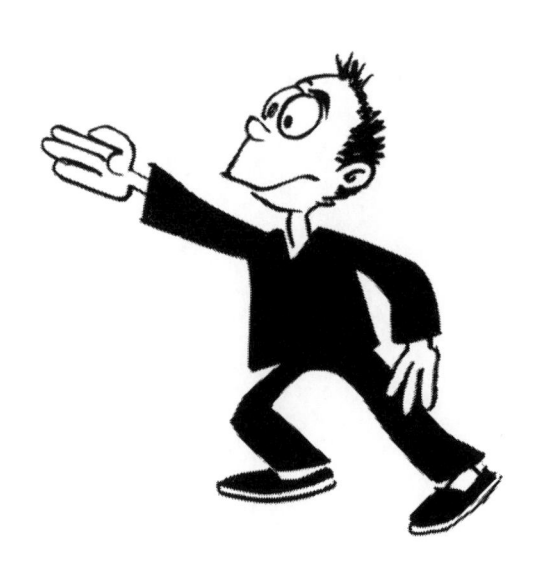

Points on Using The Principles of Tai Chi.

As most students and practitioners of Tai Chi Chuan know, the concepts that come from the "principles" are the tools which empower Tai Chi.

All practitioners, if they are performing their Tai Chi according to what we understand historically, and wish to attain the 'Kung Fu' (skill) of the art, must utilize and implement these principles.

It is our understanding of them that give us the keys to all the mental, physical, and spiritual aspects that make Tai Chi work for us.

Whether you are interested in only the martial, the health benefits, inner relaxation, or meditation you still need to adhere to these principles, which have been handed down in the classics for generations, if you wish to attain any of them or all of them.

Tai Chi is a never ending circle of learning, just when you think you have achieved your own personal excellence, a posture in the form suddenly becomes uncomfortable or just "doesn't feel right

Or maybe your push hands partner work seems to be letting you down, and you feel tension creeping back.

It is usually standard practice to apply more than one idea or concept along with a principal.

However until you have explored and are clear in your mind what the original classics are conveying, it will be difficult to attempt this.

Many of the old classic teachings refer to moving and aligning the body in a certain way. E.g. "sink the shoulders, relax the chest".

This is to let the body receive energy more easily, while relying on as little muscle power as possible. This will protect your body from as much damage as possible.

The principles are there to help practitioners understanding, but there is much more to explore apart from the written word.

We must not forget that many teachings as they moved down the years were "word of mouth" and we also need to explore these.

I look at them like sprinkling in an OXO cube to a stew.

It has lots of wonderful tasty ingredients, but the cube really enhances and adds to the flavour!

By the same token if you feel it doesn't work, you do not have to use it again.

It's all about exploring.

Some of the early teachers of Tai Chi taught in a way that they believed made their martial art movements effective.

They found out quite quickly if they had strayed too much from the traditional teachings as they found themselves on the ground, or with a bloody face.

They needed to be effective in the martial aspects of the art if they where to protect themselves from bandits and bullies.

Although Tai Chi in the West has a huge amount of people who purely practice to attain the health benefits the art is well known for, we must also realise it is a whole art embodying Yin and Yang, Hard and Soft, Male and Female.

Without the Martial, Tai Chi becomes simply another movement art, and although sometimes referred to as a "dance" its roots where initially deeply embedded in defending oneself.

The martial meanings provide character, purpose, depth and subtlety to the mood of the form.

The secret is not to get "stuck" in one or two of these principles or you may find your form is unbalanced.

You could become really competent at rooting, but forget about the upper bodies need for lightness and so find you are becoming too heavy and inflexible as a whole unit.

The other extreme is too much attention being focused on relaxation or what I like to call "the wet rag" syndrome.

Having spirit, and "peng" and the ability to have connected body structure to manifest power is sometimes lost in this situation.

I think the answer lies in not spending too much time on any one principle. Give it a few months if you are still struggling, move on to another one. You can then come back to it at a later date and find the break has given you new in site into what was going wrong.

These classic principles although forming the basis of our art, have over the centuries been added to and extended to make the understanding of them and applications work in a real situation in modern times.

If you try and fathom out the mysticism that surrounds Tai Chi, then it will remain just that, mystic. Tai Chi is real so practice in a real way and use the principles to help guide you.

Lao Tse's once said "The fundamental source is like an empty container: it can be used but never exhausted. It is like the eternal void, filled with infinite possibilities."

I have listed below one of the most comprehensive lists of Tai Chi principles that I could find without being too long
See how many you think you understand and can effectively practice, and think about the one's you need to give more thought to. (Ask your class instructor if in doubt)

1. Have slowness and Evenness
2. Use Alignment and Structure
3. Have Mindfulness and Sensitivity
4. Have Stillness in Movement.
5. Use Simultaneousness and Unity
6. Have Relaxation with Vitality
7. Use Mind –Intent with Feeling
8. Sink the Chi
9. Raise the Spirit
10. Manifest Power (natural strength)
11. Have Balance
12. Use Circularity and Flow
13. Have Rootedness below, Responsiveness above.
14. Distinguish and Harmonize Yin and Yang
15. Have softness, Fullness, and Roundness
16. Practice Regularly and Persevere.

Inside Out Martial Arts

It's often said, particularly by senior instructors, that all martial arts are the same. However, just looking at taiji begs the question, if they are all the same, why does this one look so different? Well, like all good scientists I have a theory. Having spent quite a few years now on each side of this divide, I can see a clear contrast, and it really is a question of which end of the stick you are holding. The interesting question then, is what is in the middle?

The first major principle people grasp in taiji is rooting. After that you start to learn about building a good body structure, and then you start to understand sensitivity and the flow of force between people, by practicing the eight ways and push hands. Then movements begin to take on a life of their own. More forms might be learned, perhaps weapons to help learn to extend ones power even further and to focus the intent. As you enter these later stages applications start to appear. They may not be explicitly taught, and rightly not, rather, they are noticed.

In other ancient arts the first major principle you learn is intent, the attack, then you learn to move around that attack and break your opponents balance. You learn shapes and forms that deal with such attacks. You might learn weapons to help develop intent and focus to higher levels, or you might strive to achieve this through sparring, or simply through the way you organise you're training sessions. Over time you learn more and more forms, typically partner based, and you drill them relentlessly. Over time you develop sensitivity, when a movement goes wrong you get the feeling why and you start to understand the flow of force between people. You realise that the techniques of your form are just shapes that appear in the air, they are gambits that you will follow when the opportunity comes. Good body structure has become a habit and you begin to notice that you have a strong root.

So you can see that taiji is an art that begins with the ground beneath your feet, and comes to a recognition of what can be done to deal with an attack, whereas most other arts begin with how to deal with an attack, then come to a recognition of what is possible when you make good use of the ground beneath your feet.

So what is in the middle? Feeling. It is the one common link that connects all arts; ultimately they are about how you respond in the moment, what is the feeling of the movement that you make together with your adversary? In all arts I have studied it is the same, smooth and fluid, until someone has an accident, your only job is not to be the one having the accident, or as Mark says – don't fall over.
Ben Ford – Instructor

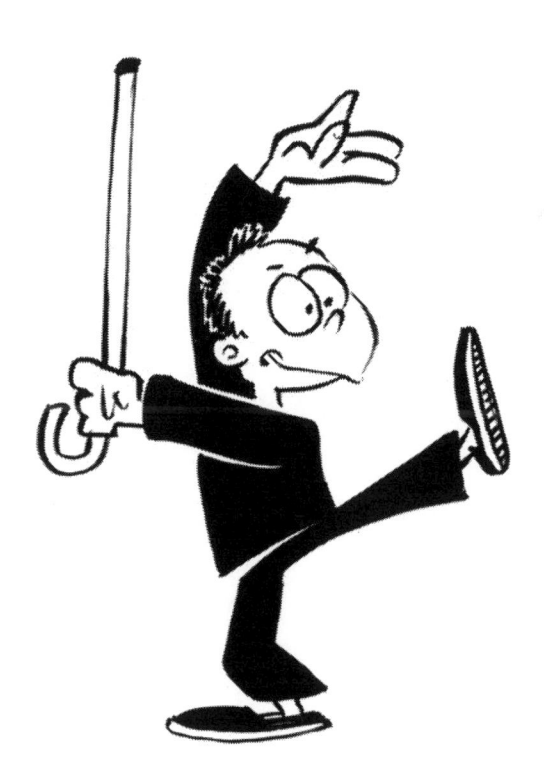

Are There Circles And Squares In Tai Chi?

In Tai Chi Chuan circular movements can be found in ALL movement, offensive, open or close; it is still circular.
This circular movement is divided into big, small, visible, invisible, horizontal, and vertical. They are either up, down, open, close, soft, hard, slow, or fast;
All done in a circular motion.
The classics "Tai Chi Chuan is circular.
It does not matter what direction. It never leaves this circle.
Tai Chi Chuan is square.
It does not matter what direction. It never leaves this square.
Circle and square interact with each other.
Square is open and circle is compact.
When one is familiar with this principle, one's practice can go beyond this principle."
The classics also point out the significance of the square and circle existing together.
"If the style is only in the circle without the square, the style is a soft fist. (INTERNAL)
If the style is only in the square without the circle, the style is a hard fist" (EXTERNAL)
All the movements in Tai Chi are continuous rotation, waist, wrist, shoulders, hips etc.
When not in motion the body stops.
The circle and square concept in Tai Chi is another interpretation of Yin and Yang
The classics also emphasize the balance of circle and square, yet all the movements are circular and not square.
Why is this? Circle refers to a circular motion.
Square refers to A STRAIGHT MOTION.
The classics state "seek the straight within the curve"
It is often said among internal arts practitioners that circular motion is for the mobilization of Qi and square is for the discharge of power.
Therefore, when a Tai Chi movement appears to be circular, if the movement can discharge power, it is already a square motion.

This is why the Tai Chi Classics say that one must square the body and focus in one direction to discharge power.

The circular motion in Tai Chi is the movement of internal power.

This internal power is mobilized by rotating inside the body up and down, left and right.

It has penetration characterized by rotation.

Anyone who uses a drill in the house will understand this theory.

When something travels in a spiral it will travel further.

The Tai Chi beginner is recommended to begin practice with large movements, later they should work with more compact movement.

It is a method to develop application techniques, for they will gradually increase ability, mobility and speed.

If they train in this way they are preparing the body to react in an instant.

When the body is nimble, agile and mobile, it all adds up to a powerful strike.

To help understand and develop these principles the following points should be paid attention to in practice.

1. Concentration; Pay attention to each movement. Find the circular motion within. As your practice and focus improves they will become more apparent.
2. Slow motion; Beginners need the slow movements initially to help them remember the postures. Also speed is harder to control.
3. Relaxation; Necessary as circular motion is based on this, we can use all our senses when relaxed.
4. Storage; be flexible. When one has to spend something, do not spend all; save something for later. We talk about storage and release. For power to be released we have to store the same amount first A circular motion involves extension and contraction in the muscle to do this.

The three major characteristics of a circle are; many shapes, very smooth, and infinite motion.

A true circular motion in Tai Chi develops the person to be flexible and nimble, with speed, mobility, and agility.

A Beginners Guide To Class Confusion

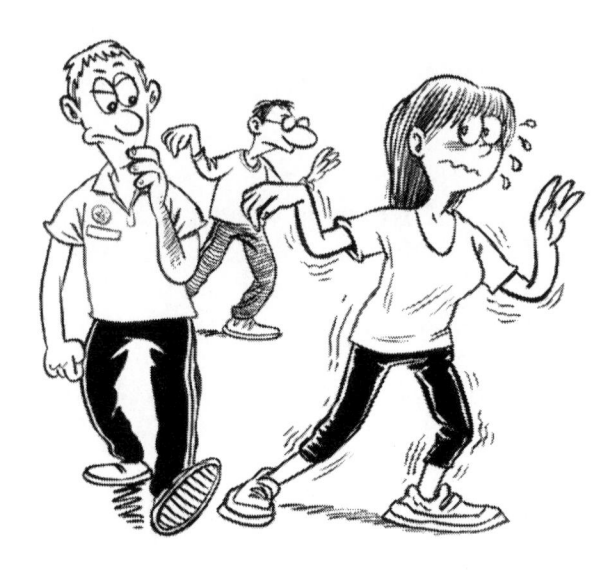

We are currently working on a new "beginners guide" but for now here are some useful points to note, compiled by Ian Anderson - Instructor

Yang Cheng Fu's 10 essentials to correct tai chi
1. Straightening the head & neck
2. Correct position of chest and back
3. Relax (loosen) the waist
4. Differentiate full and empty
5. Sinking of shoulders and elbows
6. Using the mind instead of force
7. Coordination of upper and lower parts
8. Harmony between the internal and external parts
9. Importance of continuity
10. Seek stillness in motion

COMMONLY USED terms you may hear in a class

Bai Huai point
Imagine yourself as "being suspended from above". This point is where the line between nose and spine and ears meet - dissect. The crown of the head, normally. Have a feeling of pressing the top of the head upwards. Lengthens the spine and frees middle & lower back and chest. Chin slightly in, and jaw relaxed. The main point is to loosen head and elongate the spine. This also places the head in correctly supported position. Important as it weighs approximately as much as a bowling ball.

Fair Lady's hand
Important in Cheng Man Ching Tai Chi. The hand is soft, open and relaxed. Not stretched or tense. Fingers relaxed. The hand sits on the wrist and there should not be any tension in the hand or visible on the back of the hand.

Long Quan point
Fold your middle finger so that the tip touches your palm and you find this point. You can visualise this point as connecting to the ground, feet and each hand.

Tigers mouth
Found approximately in the space (web) when your thumb and forefinger are relaxed and slightly separated.

Yong chun point
Point in centre of foot just below to ball of foot. Visualise this point relaxing and dissolving into the ground. Helps to relax feet, ankles, shins and calves

Constant Bear exercise
Key to CMC style Tai Chi practice. Teaches you about moving with correct body alignment, moving from the centre of the body, leading (and loosening) the waist (KUA), weight change, and how not to move outside your own structure.

Allows practice of relaxing muscles not used in turning and activating those that are just enough to move. .

Standing post (e.g. Lift hands, Play Guitar, Preparation,)
Allows you to develop posture and in Chinese medicine standing quietly and attentively is considered a very healthy activity for several reasons. Postures lift hands & play guitar practice 'rooting'(relaxing) through foot, ankle, shin, knee, thigh, hip/pelvis/ waist, lengthen spine etc.

Ming men point
Think of a point on the spine roughly in line with naval and practise a feeling of filling this point when you breath in.

Dantien
Very important. Just below the naval and a couple of inches inside is where your attention should be focuses in all practice. Considered to be the point where CHI (bio-energy) can be stored. Pay attention to it when you move.

Sacrum/coccyx
Essentially, the lower part of the pelvis and spine ... have a feeling (yes it's getting repetitive??) of rolling it under your bum... naturally... as it just resting gently on a high stool.

Breathing
Natural breathing - simples!!! - in through nose, out through nose, slow and easy. Just don't forget to breath. Like a balloon, let the body expand when breathing in, and deflate when breath out.

Where to look when you practise
Soften your gaze, and take in all your surroundings. Practise using peripheral vision. Because it is sensitive to movement. Look where you want to go but move your gaze and body together.

Nose lined with naval
For most moves your nose stays in line with your naval. There are exceptions (i.e. Lift hands - where your waist is 45 degrees and nose faces where you look.)

Tongue on roof of mouth
Close your mouth gently and let your tongue rest on your upper pallet. This aids release of saliva (in TCM saliva has a healing quality) and relaxes the throat.

Chi – bio-energy
Life force (Skywalker's - Force), bio-energy essentially. Practising the form helps release energy around the body and can assist with health in various ways.

Sink chest - pluck the back
This means simply to relax the shoulders down naturally, and allow the chest to drop down (as opposed to a soldier standing to attention with chest thrown forward, shoulder blades pulled in towards each other). Don't slump or collapse though.

Sung
See above. There is no real translation but the closest possible is relaxed and alive. A state of readiness, liveliness and alert in both mind and body.

Fear - relaxation – (less fear – more relaxation, etc etc)
Fear has a lot of disguises and is also very natural. If we didn't feel fear we would not survive as a race. However, the fears we face have changed for instance from Sabre tooth tigers to incompetent bankers, from searching for firewood to stressing (a fear disguise) about paying the bill for the heating! Same feelings, different cause.

Tai Chi helps to relax mind and body which can lessen the feeling of fear and help you to be aware of the " thousand faces of fear" when it comes knocking. Our martial practice develops from a point of relaxation, and gets more relaxed... become a peaceful warrior.

There Is No Transition

Do you remember those pre Tai Chi days when you used to get in your car or walk down the high street, and all of a sudden you were at your destination! The transition (or as I prefer to call it – the Journey) was 'lost'. You missed the whole journey, experience, that's part of your valuable life – your mind was 'somewhere else', or 'a blank', or focused on the end of the journey.

Whatever 'valid' reason you came up with – you missed the journey – you were basically not in full control, not with it, not consciously aware, not mindful, and not living in the second.

The same can be said (sometimes) of the macro level too – "don't the weeks, year's wiz by".

With Tai Chi we have all learned to be present, mindful and aware.

So when doing the form (say) I now never think/feel I am moving from one 'position' to another. As every second, every sub-second, of that journey is a unique flow. Sometimes both feet are on the ground – but always feeling the ground more with one foot than the other, always moving, sometimes one foot on the ground and the other off the ground, always feeling aligned with gravity.

But never stagnate, never stuck, never not moving - however slowly, however little the move. So I try and feel every sub-second as its own unique movement along that 5, 10, 15 minute continually following journey.

There is no transition – it is all a continual journey to be enjoyed.

Tai Chi And The Element Of Relaxation.
How / Why / When?

The ability to relax, muscles, mind, etc is a natural inheritance. We are born with it, but unfortunately as we grow our view of life and our need to pursue various new avenues (sometimes too vigorously) we leave behind this very necessary commodity

In its most simple form, because we are striving to survive in a sometimes "mad" world, or gain acceptance, or be as good or better than others in our circle we cannot find or make time to relax, or think "there will be plenty of time to do that later".

Tai Chi can give you back that ability, and the focus to achieve it.

The relaxation of mind, body, and spirit (emotions) that you can find in this art goes way beyond sitting on the sofa watching TV with a cup of tea (as nice as that may be).

When muscles and joints are relaxed that do not work against each other, they release pressure off the veins and arteries. This allows the blood flow through them that carries the oxygen to the heart and major organs etc, and the impurities and waste that needs to be recycled through liver and kidneys to function more efficiently.

The brain also has an increased oxygen supply aiding the thought process, and hopefully the "feel good factor" will kick in more frequently when the stresses of outside influences can be left behind while we practice our form or a Chi-Kung set.

We do not just stretch an arm or a leg or joint, but the entire body as we practice.

The body has been likened to a bow in archery by some, or even many bows throughout the body that are activated in Tai Chi practice.

In drawing a bow, there is a stretching that requires relaxing and at the same time tension.

When the arrow is released, the bow and the bowstring are released and lose certain vibrancy.

The stretching in Tai Chi Chuan occurs vertically, horizontally, circularly.

For instance, in the torso there is a pulling upward by the lifting of the top of the head and lifting the back.

At the same time, there is a pulling downward at the base of the spine, which creates traction for a healthy and flexible back.
When the arm is extended, it stretches outward, but by sinking the elbow and settling the shoulders, there is a counter stretch.

This kind of stretching can be seen in the silk reeling action, which involves a spiral twisting in the arms, legs, and torso by "relaxed" positive, counter stretches that feel like squeezes.

The stretches are the Yang counterpoint of the Yin relaxation.

A good way to envisage the kind of relaxation that Tai Chi uses is to think of the relaxed nature of water. It is soft, changeable, and also powerful.

Its power is derived in part from the way it is contained, for example, by a dam or river bank.

Imagine a sealed plastic bag filled with water, you can see the fluidity of the water and how it reacts when it is squeezed, trying to move to another location, with force when the force is strong. Yet it is always true to its relaxed nature.

The human body contains many fluids and as we move we are exerting a certain amount of force on them as in Tai Chi.
However, if we are tense in many local places, the fluids are blocked from their natural flow and can even stagnate; we only need to look to respiratory and circulatory problems to see this. Cheng Man Ching's focus on Sung (relaxed, alive and pliable) is key to this as is differentiating Yin and Yang…

Yang Style Tai Chi Chuan Twenty-Character Motto

- Excerpt from Yang Zhenduo, Yang Shih Taiji, 1997

> 楊氏太極拳二十字口訣
> (附上級繁术)
> 抻出肘尖；空出腋肢窩。
> 肘尖拽膀尖、連手腕帶手指

"Extend the elbows outward; leave a hollow in the armpits. The elbows pull down the tops of the shoulders, connect the wrists and carry along the fingers."

The Twenty-Character Motto is very brief, yet its meaning is very profound and worth pursuing.

Although only the various parts of the upper limbs are mentioned, following this motto can set in motion a chain of causality in which changes here affect the other parts of the body. This connection is not just mental, but you can actually feel that precisely this movement of the upper limbs causes you to 'hold the chest in', which in turn induces 'pulling up the back', leading to 'relaxation of waist and hips' and ultimately bringing about '(movement proceeds) from feet to legs to waist', so 'all the joints are working interconnected as a whole'.

You can get an internal sensation of the integration of all these principles and how they support each other.

The sense of energy created by this, and the sensation of the whole-body working together are things which every player must work toward and actually experience. This is crucial to successfully learning taiji. From this we can see that the Twenty-Character motto separately relates to every individual posture of taiji and as a whole determines the connected completion of the entire form.

I hope that students will diligently seek to understand this, and experience the 'sensation of energy' induced by this 'extend', 'hollow', 'pull down', and 'connect'. This will aid your overall level of training as well as the practice of connecting the internal and external

The Riddle of the Tai Chi Classics

'How many Tai Chi teachers does it take to change a light bulb?'

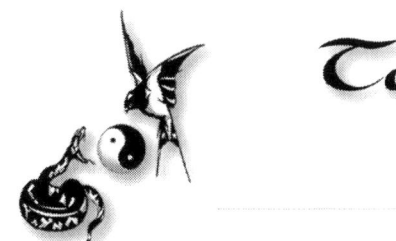

We have all done riddles.

Sometimes you can puzzle for ages to get the answer. Once you realise, it is so obvious that you know it is the right answer.

The tai chi classics are like riddles. You have to put the work in, then one day you realise: 'That's what it means'.

You can read them over and over again looking for their meanings to no avail. In fact the harder you look, the less you will see.

If you practice every day, once in a while a glorious 'Oh!' moment will occur. Then it is so obvious, You think: 'Why didn't I see that before.'

I remember discussing this with my teacher, He said 'The classics are so annoying they mean exactly what they say but you can't figure them out.'

They are more like marker posts along a path so that you know you have not wandered off into the wilderness. They are always carefully placed just round a bend or hidden behind a bush so that you only know that you have found one when you stumble across it. There is no seeing it in the distance and working towards the goal.

Happily a teacher cannot give you the answers; all they can do is encourage you towards them. Why happily? Well if you were given the answers, the joy of the 'Oh!' moment would be lost and the answer not treasured.

By the way the answer is:
Just one, but there are a hundred others watching who say: "That's very good, but in our style it's much nicer if you do it like this..."

The importance of Dong-Dang (swing-return)

Dong-Dang is a concept at the core of Cheng Man Ching's tai chi; it is the process that creates a loose momentum when practicing tai chi

It is interesting to analyze the two words in Chinese character.

"Dong" is formed by two characters: weight and force, pronounced in mandarin, zhong li which means in English "gravity", functioned by the pull of the earth.

"Dang" is consisted of two words, "soup" in the "bowl"; the soup symbolizes flexibility like water. While the soup in the bowl in your hand is in motion, you can feel the gravity and the water soup swinging freely and at will. It is easy to feel outside object in your hand, but hard to feel one's inside with this sign if one can't be relaxed, soft and can't feel one's own hanging weight.

Master Cheng's New Method of Tai chi Chuan Self-Cultivation", translator Mark Hennessy refers to this as to "momentate." Page XI: "Every movement, according to Cheng, produces momentum. And the true secret to a smooth-flowing tai chi form is to redirect momentum back to movement - which produces more movement and momentum." This brings the question of form speed to mind.... Practicing slowly is beneficial for many reasons but slowly is a word an open to your own interpretation. Natural sits better for me as it allows changes in speed to suit the feel and flow of each of us as individuals and implies no speed fast or slow.

Play with the idea and play with your form to see what this brings out for you...

The Waist And its Importance in Tai Chi Practice.

(A) Look at the physiological structure of the human body.
The spine can transmit strength and keep adjusting all movements so they are not out of balance.
It lies in the centre of the back of the body and is a pivot of a trunk, made up with a central core and an elastic cartilage plate between each vertebra.
Normal spinal functions in sports depend on the inflation of the inner core of the vertebra, because when the spine moves, the core can change the way the form moves at any time, thus increasing the range of movement.
This proves that the thickness of the vertebra determines the spines range of activity.
A study of anatomy shows the vertebras in the waist area are made up of five vertebrae.
The alternate thickness (vertical height) in the middle is 11.3 mm. 11.4 mm. 14.8 mm 17.1 mm. respectively.
Secondly, the chest area has the minimum of only a little more than two mm in vertical height. So it is with good grounds that the waist is the most flexible and the activity range is the largest.

(B) Examine the position of the waist;
By anatomy, the waist lays in the body's trunk, above the joint of the hip, under two soft ribs. It has the pubic region in front.
It is believed in Chinese martial arts the qi that is stored and distributed throughout the body all comes from the pubic area in which lies the "dan-tian"
It is necessary for the human body to be fully relaxed, waist and abdomen especially so that the qi can sink inward and gather there. (Loosening and sinking)
In order to prevent practicing with the waist arching so the buttocks protrude to form a concave, the waist must be straightened.
This straightening allows you to be able to carry and pull. Loosening and sinking also indicates that the hip pivot is rotated and the waist is not curved, not swayed and is straight.

Because the whole body is relaxed, all the weight above the waist is secured by the waist. So if you want to be strong, the waist must be straight. No pitching forward or back, or left to right.

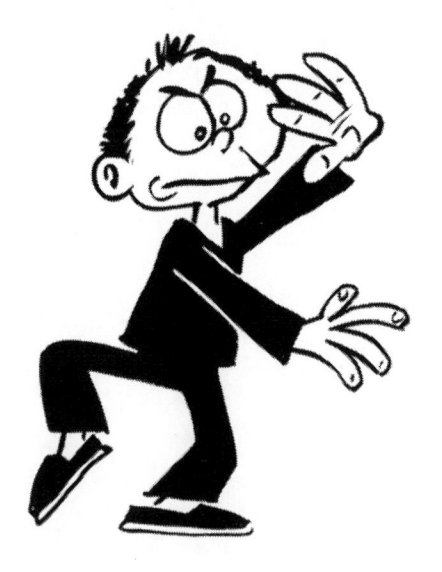

The Inner Game

When the mind is free of any thought or judgement, it is still and acts like a perfect mirror. Then and only then can we know things as they are.
W. Timothy Gallway.

I remember being told many years ago that it takes at least 20 years to master tai chi, and I guess they meant have a reasonable understanding of because mastery is such a subjective term. But why should it take any longer than any other martial art or any other skill for that matter? Nigel Sutton always said the only secret was practice and I would only add to this by saying mindful practice. For me this is the Inner Game as discussed by Timothy Gallway in his great book.

I became interested in NLP (neuro-linguistic programming) after Jenny mentioned it in connection to management of change but I never realised where it would lead…..
I started learning NLP for work and found new perspectives on my tai chi training. The description given by its co-developer Richard Bandler is 'the study of the structure of subjective experience' and at the core of it is 'the map is not the territory' or 'the word is not the thing', Alfred Korzybski. What this all means is that we map our experiences and measure against them so are constantly making unconscious judgements/decisions, some good some not. I mention all this because it seems what has made Tai Chi more difficult to grasp, beyond the basic shapes, is you have to get your head out of the way, to suspend reality for a moment and just experience the experience as it unfolds. Sounds a bit heavy I know but then reality is not real, the map is not the territory remember. Have you ever seen the Wizard of Oz? (the original version not the remake); near the end when they're all in front of the great wizard asking for courage, a heart, a brain etc. they notice something and the wizards said "Pay no attention to the man behind the curtain". The whole story is a great metaphor for what I am discussing because the man behind the curtain is your unconscious mind, pulling the strings, doing all the work.

I hope I haven't bored you and that I still have your attention because luckily there is a solution and that is called mindful practice or as Tim Gallway said "when the mind is still". Even the tai chi classis state "Only motion attained through stillness may be called Tai Chi". But here is the dilemma, how to practice stillness without being still because tai chi is an art of feel and flow…

A phrase I like is 'you're only limited by your own creativity' or to paraphrase NLP 'you're only limited by your own map limits'. I have found dropping the names of things (remember the word is not the thing) and making games up to develop your own experience of things can be both fun and shorten the learning cycle. Once you realise the old adage "if you keep at it, you'll get it in the end" needs a rethink because if you keep doing what you've always done, you'll keep getting what you've always got. I know, I know…. I'm starting to sound like a range of t-shirt quotes but hey, they can be helpful!

Anyway, back to it… Diligent practice, mindful practice, reflective practice is what makes the difference and so tai chi should only take as long as it takes to quiet disbelief. Be clear on what you want from it, have a well-formed outcome, and train with that in mind. And remember the best part is the journey – your classes and your own practice. Quiet the chatter and enjoy the inner game.

Q&A From Huang Sheng-Shyan (Huang Xingxian)

HIGH OR LOW STANCE IN THE TAIJIQUAN FORM?

Within the art of Taijiquan there is no distinction between high and low postures, but is rather based on the idea of 4 "balances" or equilibriums:
1. Balance in the magnitude of the posture or movement, such as both sides of the body must have "balanced" amounts of spatial displacement (expansion in all directions) when moving;
2. Accuracy/precision - achieved simultaneously by all parts of the body;
3. Bodily balance when moving or turning;
4. Steadiness particularly when moving.

External and internal balance or harmony must be cultivated so there is no slanting of the central axis of the body. When jin (energy) is needed the bent back knee will move up or straighten slightly, though the height of the body remains unchanged. This is so yi (mind-intent) and chi can 'close' centrally, instead of coming up while the bent knee is used to adjust accordingly.

The yi is used to lead the muscles in relaxing. Joints, muscles, and ligaments must then be loosened, relaxed, and "thrown" open, but still be linked.

The body is then erect and comfortable. Yi is also used to 'move' Taijiquan principles to all parts of the body. Having achieved the four balances the question of high and low postures is then answered through mindful feedback when practicing taijiquan (Tai Chi Chuan).

To expand on this, low stances in taiji can be more cardio-vascular but can also break the principles of looseness and relaxation so it is essential to practice with a clear goal in mind i.e. aerobic workout or sung (relaxed balance).

Through regular attentive (mindful) practice you will develop a natural flow and stance; Taiji, in technical terms, is a sophisticated form of whole body Neuromuscular/skeletal movement re-education. With good use, the body moves easily - with balance and coordination; both mental and physical; it develops proprioception and kinaesthesia which are essential for everyday life.

Cheng man Ching is often quoted as responding to the question "when do my legs stop aching?" with "when you stop improving". With this in mind, stances should be low and loose enough to work/activate the relevant muscles enough, yet high enough to still move freely and in-balance.

Explore what the 4 balances mean to you and if in doubt, ask!

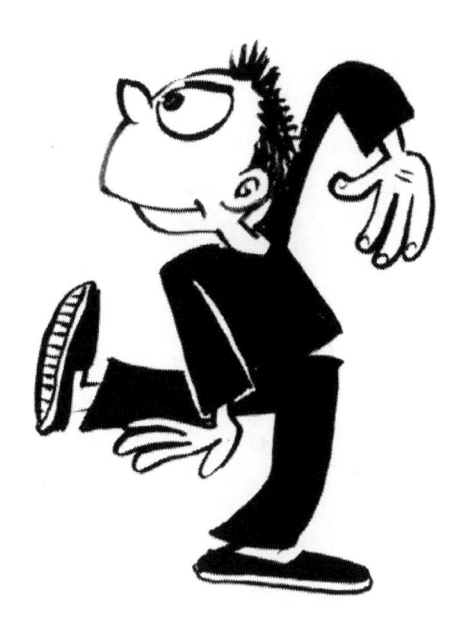

The Importance Of The Five Loosening Exercises
From Master Huang Sheng Shyan.
By Master Willie Lim

As exponents of the 37, from the Lineage of GM Cheng Man-Ching, the form needs to be looked at with an acute eye. Many an exponent thinks that learning the form means they are on the way there??! On the way there but how far ahead. little do people realise that within the 37 moves are hidden the 108. Where I am often asked? I change and mould as I move along the form that must be refined and refined. How do I go about this? Master Huang has left us the five loosening exercises that with proper execution of them, and knowing where they fit into the form, we can refine the form and move ahead in the 37. What do the loosening exercises involve? The Chinese translation is "Hue-Shou" meaning throwing hands, hence you get lead astray if you interpret as such."Throwing hand" is just a simple phrase to describe the refinement that must go into the exercises when you perform them. The best way to understand how these exercise are performed is to look at two different analogies. Take rhythmic gymnastics where the girl plays with the ribbon; that is Tai chi at its best. The line you have to remember here is the girl never moves the ribbon. The next analogy is the weightlifter cleaning the weight. What is common here? Both are identical muscle activities. How do you relate one to the other and where are they the same? The same sequential motion of the muscles are in play. This is what you have to look for when training the 5 loosening exercises, so they in turn fit into the 37 and refine the form. I believe today that without understanding these exercise one cannot develop "ting jing" or listening energy. Differentiate the straight from the curve, full and empty, connect and disconnect, torque and compression. These are some of the principals that are involved.

Take the rotation exercise or No.1 - What is involved? How do you differentiate the straight from the curve here? When is one arm full and the other empty. Does the body and the arm move at the same time? What are the joints that have to be lined up when one sits into one side? How is the arm 'brought' up and how it is let 'down'. Do I really move the arm? When does the caving of the body come in? Do I really cave in or do a "counter rotation cave in" (sink the chest, pluck the back). Where does the compression and the torque come in? There is more and more I could go on.....

This is how you have to look at the loosening exercise and in turn fit them in to your form to really move on. Tai chi is based on simple principles that have to be honed into the body. It is never easy because it needs time and guidance from someone who is ahead of you to guide you along that path. Just look at master Huang on YouTube. Look at other tai chi Masters. Do they even ever come close to him? For your information master Huang is the one who taught the founder of Goju karate. Tai chi is a journey which is full of twist and turn. It is not as many think, collecting forms, while that has its place as well. Be critical of every small change and enjoy the journey, because it is a lifetime's work moulded into the 37.

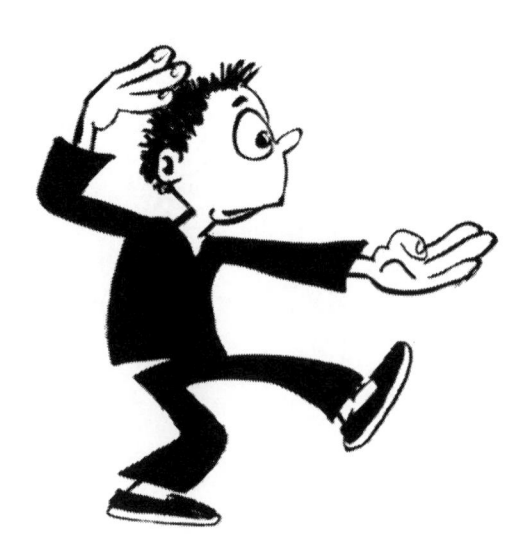

Q&A From Huang Shengshyan (Huang Xingxian)

How should we practice taijiquan (Tai Chi Chuan) in order to reach accuracy?
The gap between accurate and non-accurate achievement is wide. Remember the words of the
ancient Taijiquan master Wang Zongyue, that the body must be naturally and vertically balanced, and that one must bear in mind the principles of being relaxed, rounded, and aware of the various parts of the body. During practice of the form, one must be careful, conscious or alert, observant, and must feel where one is moving. Otherwise there is form without substance and deception of others. To achieve accuracy, the principles of Taijiquan must be followed, in addition to having correct methods of practice. A good master is necessary, coupled with one's own constant research. The art must be learned progressively; one must be on firm ground first, before advancing to the next step. Personal requirements are also important. One must be determined, confident, persevering, and motivated. One must have a secure means of livelihood and a normal environment; these, coupled with learning and practice, and a clear, thorough understanding of the principles—all this will lead to achievement of accuracy. This is in contrast to those who want to learn fast, who concern themselves with the external forms and who learn and practice sporadically. Those who hope to learn first and be corrected later do not realize that this is worse than having a new person learn from scratch. Others take the principles of Taijiquan lightly or superficially and liken the art to a common exercise, drill, or dance.

All of these cases have form but no substances. One's body must be likened to a perfect machine where a wrong spare part will affect the operation of the machine. The founder of Taijiquan said, "achieving the Dao is important, acquiring skill in the art is secondary; but not learning my Dao, he is not my student". Therefore, also important are honesty, righteousness, and a good moral character.

For me this question and answer explains the importance of mindful practice without the distractions of life's daily worries, impatience or aims of self-aggrandisation. Once these are removed from the equation then the body and mind can focus on developing the inner skills of taijiquan (Tai Chi Chuan) or as Willie calls it 'moulding into the form'. Steven Covey is often quoted as saying "begin with the end in mind" which can be applied here as 'practice with intention', what is your aim? To feel natural balance, to play the postures and see where they lead, to discover martial possibility, accuracy, to…. Well, whatever you choose! As GM Cheng says "form without function is no form at all". This does not mean just fighting; it too means what is your aim! To practice without intention is to play an empty dance; the classics are a guidebook of intentions you can play with as are Huang's 5 loosening exercises. Accuracy is not an outside shape it's an inside feel; when the feel is right the shape and application becomes naturally correct. The advanced monthly classes I run aren't about learning new forms or techniques; they are about developing a deeper practical understanding of tai chi (Taijiquan) as a living art. What is your aim? You can change it by the way, as you no doubt will as you train more and more. An aim gives you the ability to develop accuracy, well how can you be accurate if you don't know what you're striving to be accurate at!

The wonderful things is once you have planned your journeys end (the aim) you are free to enjoy the journey and discoveries made along the way.

Q&A From Huang Sheng-Shyan (Huang Xingxian)

How can substantiality and insubstantiality be distinguished between left and right or between top and bottom parts of the body?

Answer: The muscles, the skeleton, and the nerves are parts of the body system. When practicing movements, the use of consciousness to sink and relax the body is most important. The centre of gravity is moved while preserving the uprightness of the central axis of the body. It is important to focus on steadiness, tranquillity, relaxation, and rootedness. The internal movements propel the external movements in a continuous or uninterrupted fashion. Internal force is generated with turning movements. After a long time, the whole body is in balance. When left and right is distinguished, one is substantial and the other insubstantial along the pattern of "cross alignment." For example, together with the distinction between top and bottom parts of the body, when the left upper part of the body is substantial, the left lower part is insubstantial and similarly when the right upper part of the body is substantial, the right lower part is insubstantial.

This pattern of cross alignment (cross-pumping) is used in shifts of the centre of gravity from one leg to the other. This is similar to the "cross-roads" of the nervous system. When moving chi, therefore, one must separate substantial from insubstantial, move the step without moving the body or moving the body and not the hand. If in moving a step, the body also moves, then it is not separating substantial from insubstantial. If in moving the body, the hand also moves, then the shoulder and the hands are not relaxed.

It is important to follow the principles of using consciousness to propel movement. The top and bottom, left and right portions of the body must be coordinated. A rounded grinding stone may move but the centre is not moving. All the parts of the body become one system characterized by lightness and agility, roundness and smoothness, even respiration, alternate opening and closing like that of the sea where with movement from one part of the sea, all parts are also moved. The movements are guided by consciousness and are properly regulated like the regular movements of the waves in the sea.

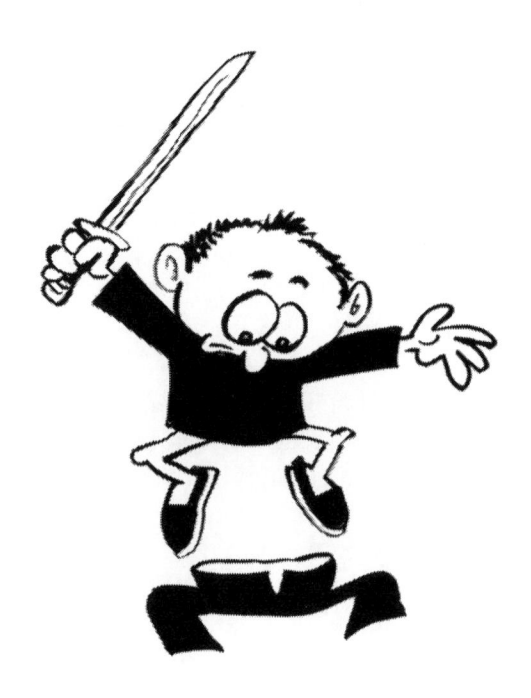

By distinguishing full and empty I am able to make contact with you but you will be unaware of any part, except the point of contact, until it hits you square in the face! What I mean by this is that if the point of contact is substantial then everything else is unsubstantial. If we continue to use the analogue of the sea as Huang has above then let's look at another of my favourite sayings by Morihei Ueshiba, "if you strike flowing water it leaves no hole". There are no gaps or hollows, there is no push or pull just a natural flow of insubstantial to substantial. Being able to differentiate means that everything flows in behind and continues the flow without a noticeable change; some people call this lightness or sensitivity I prefer the word constant as there is no change. Tai Chi as an art does not hack whether empty hand or weapon, it glides through where it meets no resistance because it knows how to separate substantial from insubstantial – it does not meet substantial with substantial (force with force) or visa-versa, it knows they go hand in hand like an elegant dance. Refining the chain reaction through the body is one of the greatest treasures Huang gave us with the 5 loosening exercises; look for the full and empty, open and closed in every stage. Peter Ralston says "hand up you down" where the hand is substantial and everything else is insubstantial. Willie Lim says "know the 50-50" which is the cross-roads of substantial and insubstantial. As you push a door what is what? As you pick something up what is what? As you touch swords what is what? How do we connect without snatching or bumping? Be like sifu silver-ball and contact at all points and resist at none. When you meet substantial with insubstantial it can find no ground; when it becomes insubstantial you take it! Look to your form and play with natural flow as going to fast or to slow cannot differentiate.

Q&A From Huang Sheng-Shyan (Huang Xingxian)

Question: Some students have been learning and practicing Tai Chi for several years and are yet unstable. Why is this so?

Answer: A lot of students are using wrong learning and practicing technique. Students must start with understanding the Tao or philosophy, then the principles, then using the correct method and finally putting in the effort. He must understand the relationship of man and his surroundings or the universe and use the method of chi to practice. He must be humble and persistent in his practice. Slowly, rootedness will result and the method of practicing is understood. Understand the principles and be aware of the less obvious and unnoticeable aspects in slowing acquiring skill. Being rooted and having internal force can never be observed externally. They can be accomplished

through correct method. In practicing the movement and developing the internal force, the joints of the body must be loosened and yet linked. The whole body is relaxed and is not easily pushed over by an opponent. Substantiality is distinguished from insubstantiality. Aim to be flexible and pliable like a snake whose tail will come in to help if you attack the head, or vice versa or whose tail and head will assist when the centre is attacked. Be responsive to consciousness (or intent), then tranquillity and pliability can be achieved. It is easier to lift off a 200 katies iron rod than to lift up a 100 katies iron chain. This illustrates the principles of thoroughly relaxed joints. Students must also understand the application of yin and yang in the movements and push hand exercises. Yin and Yang principles are in Tai Chi which encompasses the universe: all movements whether divided according to upper and lower body, right and left, front and back, internal and external must not deviate from the principles of substantiality and insubstantiality. Moving and stillness alternate continuously: Yin does not part from Yang and vice versa. When Yang moves, Yin also moves and vice versa. This principle must be understood when practicing the set movements.

The body and the character is trained together as is the acquisition of the Tao and the art. Tao is likened to yin while the art or skill is the yang. Yang is evolved from yin and yin's completion. Being relaxed, stillness and being rooted become yin components. Neutralization of force forms the basic foundation where no strength is used. Stillness is like that of the mountain. No change is seen but it is capable of a lot of changes. The founder has said, "Tao is the basis, art is consequential." One must therefore acquire Tao by learning not to resist, for only then will the body learn to be obedient. In attacking and defending, one must understand the method, and then acquire insubstantiality and quietude. Only then will the defence be solid. Attacking will also be successful as one is naturally comfortable. In pushing hands exercise, one must learn to achieve non-resistance and stickiness. Having achieved stickiness, then one can achieve the ability to neutralize force. With adequate reserves, the neutralizing ability is applied with an involuntary exertion of internal force.

Low Punch (the lowdown)

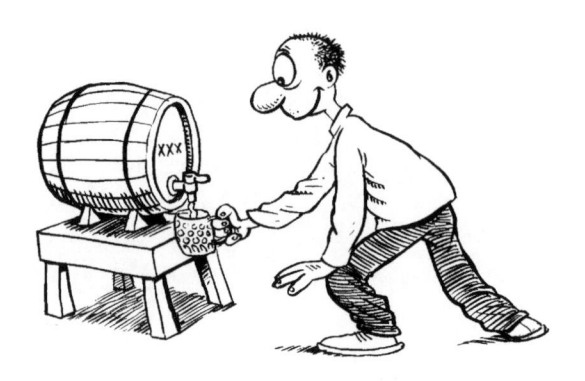

LOW PUNCH

This posture is rarely looked at and rarely well-practiced. The first group of difficulties encountered in Low Punch are related to the root. The tendency is to lean forward and pull up out of the root when doing the punch, and then at the transition out of the Low Punch, the tendency is to use the pelvis and tailbone as the axis for straightening up, rather than making use of the root in the foot.

The first scenario gives the opponent the opportunity to lead you forward out of your stance, and the latter offers an opening for him or her to apply a "ti-fang" or uproot.

The second major group of Low Punch problems is to be found in mis-angled manoeuvres; for example, an incorrect perception of the target.

In the Low Punch, just as in the horizontal punch, the target is straight ahead toward the midline of the opponent's body. The lowering and angling of the body in Low Punch should not change this target; it has simply lowered it, and it is still straight ahead of one's midline.

The Low Punch stance is also compromised by many in an effort to attain some misconceived position. Regardless of the details of this move, the stance is identical to the upright punch, with adjustments only to the angle of the torso and the amount of bend in the knees. However, one should keep both the feet flat on the ground, no matter what.

Postural alignment is a main problem area in this move, if one examines drawings, photographs and videotapes of seasoned practitioners, one will discern a great variety of positions for the peak of this punch. The majority of these practitioners appear to follow some simple guidelines:

1. Make sure that the spine does not curl, and that the head keeps in line with the spine.
Many people, without realizing it, hunch over as they do the Low Punch. Many people execute the move as if they are bowing in obedience; and in their hands the Low Punch becomes a gesture of submission, rather than a martial arts application. They raise their shoulders, tuck their heads, and curl the spine forwards.
Whether this is because of a misinterpretation of instructions or simply how they habitually bend over is difficult to ascertain. To do the move in this way is tantamount to preparing to launch a forward somersault. One becomes poised, ready to be uprooted. In an actual fight, this obviously would give the opponent a tremendous advantage. Ben Clarke once said it is as if your body is a drawing pin where your arm is the pin and your body is the head; the head pushes the pin in and must be correctly aligned so it doesn't bend or break. Ben is my tai chi senior and teaches in London.

2. Keep the eyes aware.
Simply because there is a lean forward, it does not mean that one's attention to surroundings should drop away. To do so would be like doing two tasks at the same time. One must maintain a full awareness and not let it drop away along with dropping into a lower position.

3. Lean where required by the form, but do so without compromising other principles.
Rooting is of primary importance in Taijiquan. Therefore in the Low Punch, or any time that one is required to lean, the lean forward should be done by maintaining the root, not by being too stiff, nor too limp. If one is able to keep the centre of gravity low, the root will be maintained.
The move should feel as solid as any other move in the form.

The image of the untipable (weeble) doll may be helpful; when pushed over, its innate nature is to stay connected to its root and return to an upright position.

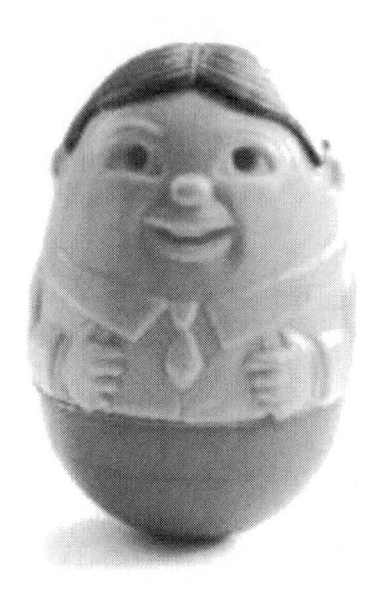

Getting it right

Recently at a class somebody made a comment about getting the level of instruction correct for the people in the group and it made me consider what is it that draws people to learning tai chi and what is it that makes a good teacher?
You may think on the face of it that a good tai chi has to have an in-depth knowledge of the art, an ability to answer virtually all questions without hesitation, to be able to spot the errors and quickly make corrections, to be beyond reproach in the quality of their own tai chi and so on…

From my perspective, I have not found this to be true; for me a good teacher: inspires you to want to learn, they don't teach answer but lead a student to discover their own answers, they identify expectations in both the student and themselves and understands that it can be those expectations that hold us back. If you are a teacher for a moment, ask yourself what are you teaching by your actions? Compliance, art-by-rote, that learning is difficult or are you teaching constant curiosity, learning can be fun, for what purpose? As a student what is your inner teacher (you) teaching you as the same rules apply.

I love the term **'pacing expectations'** as for me it means 'getting in step with' the expectations of myself and whoever I am working with. I always ask myself **"For what purpose?"** this ensures the training has an intention even if the intention is **HAVE FUN.**

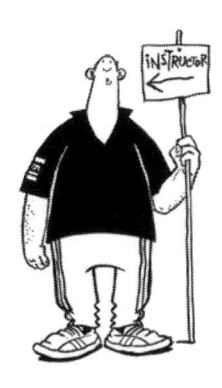

Q&A On Tao Of Tai Chi Chuan. By Master Huang Sheng Shyan

Is it better to practice Tai Chi more frequently or less frequently?

Answer: There are no extremes in Tai Chi. the essence is in the training method. If the method is not correct, it is no different from ordinary drills with a lot of time spent but relatively little achievement. So it is not a question of practicing more or less frequently but practicing correctly. That is, the central equilibrium must be vertically maintained. Every movement must be disciplined such that the posture is vertically balanced. The principles remain unchanged: There is straightness in a curve and vice versa. There must be constant learning and practice, understanding the principles and the less obvious points. Mastery of this will produce skill naturally. There is no question, therefore, of practicing too much or too little but rather of practicing correctly.

This feeds back to my opening moments in the newsletter "for what purpose practice?" Practice with awareness, Practice will intention, practice with an open heart and an open mind (Kai-ming). Better to practice once with purpose than practice one-thousand times just to say you have.

The Empowering Principles of Tai Chi

(An interesting look at their wider origin)

It is the concepts that come from within the principles of Tai Chi that enable us to become informed empowered practitioners of the art.

They have been handed down through generations of Master's who believed they were the essence of the energies and movements that give us unique properties of the form that work for health and fighting ability.

Members of the Chen and Yang families where adamant about following the principles properly.

Anyone who has been fortunate enough to study with a first generation legitimate heir to the Yang or Chen family teachings is very lucky, for as everyone knows, the more one moves away from the heart of the teachings, the more the teachings become lost.

Some variation may be good, as it can expand the approaches, concepts and ways we look at the art; but we must take care not to lose the original meanings.

Here is a list of 16 principles that have been compiled, which seem quite clear and easy to interpret.

1. Have slowness and evenness.
2. Use alignment and structure.
3. Have mindfulness and sensitivity.
4. Have stillness in movement.
5. Use simultaneousness and unity.
6. Have relaxation with vitality.
7. Use min-intent with feeling.
8. Sink the chi
9. Raise the spirit
10. Manifest power
11. Have balance
12. Use circularity and flow
13. Have root below, responsiveness above
14. Distinguish and harmonize Yin & Yang
15. Have softness, fullness, and roundness
16. Practice regularly and persevere.

This list covers all the classical principles as passed down and also includes some others that have become established over the years as important ideas.
For example the ideas of "relax" and "slowness".

Relax is mentioned by Wang Tsung-Yueh. He says the body should be erect and "relaxed", but there are very few if any other references to the idea of "relax" in any of the Yang family writings. Only that the body should be light and sensitive.
The idea of relax in general is not in Yang Cheng-Fu's principles only "relax the waist"
Relax nor slowness is not mentioned in the classic writing ascribed to Cheng San-Feng or in the Yang family manuscripts aside from Wang Tsung-Yueh
"Evenness" and "Flow" are the same things as "continuity" in the teaching of Yang Cheng-Fu and his family teachings

The power from Tai Chi may be through correct alignment of the body and movement flow and continuity, it may be practiced slowly to allow for good focus whilst training, but if for example we videoed you performing a posture in class and then played it back speeded up, the movement should look like a real application.
The full flavour of Tai Chi is found within its Martial roots, without them we are just performing another movement art.
Although the early masters and practitioners wanted to cultivate good health and mentality, they also venerated the martial side as providing character, purpose, history, .beauty and depth.
Always remember "balance" is the key word, too much time spent on trying to master one principle e.g. relaxation, applications, may result in stagnation.
If you haven't mastered it in a reasonable length of time then something may be misunderstood. Seek advice to approach it from another angle.

Many of the writings and sayings of the old Taoist Masters can be seen within Tai Chi principles.

Lao Tse and other old Taoist sages speak of stillness within the movement, and in the Taoist book of 5000 words it is written "The substantial is the root of the insubstantial; the still is the master of what moves." (Inner calm in the midst of acting in the world)

Lao Tse also said, "The wise rule without forcing; they move in accord with the times."

Is this not very like the Tai Chi teachings of "don't use force against force; let the mind lead; become one with movements."

We have all been told to "invest in loss" at some point in our training. How do we see that working in reality? Do we gain by being beaten? Do we have to lose to learn by our mistakes? Probably!

Once again we look to Lao Tse who said "For wholeness, find the partial; for forthrightness, find the unbiased; for fullness, know emptiness; for growth find loss"

In Tai Chi there is a saying "to yield is to advance; the defence is in the attack; use the

Force of four ounces to overcome great obstacles".

Again Lao Tse seems to have captured this theory by saying "Yield and overcome.

If one can give up everything, all will be given.

Why not take another look at the Taoist book of 5000 words which was attributed to him.

See how many sayings contained within its pages that seem to relate to the art of Tai Chi and its principals.

It could be an enlightening read.

Some information in this piece taken from an article in an American magazine PUBLISHED IN 1997
by Eo Omwake a teacher in Chadds Ford USA.

Dance to the Beat of Tai Chi

Just before Christmas last year I used some tai chi principles in real life for the first time. I'm happy to say it was in the gentlest of ways.

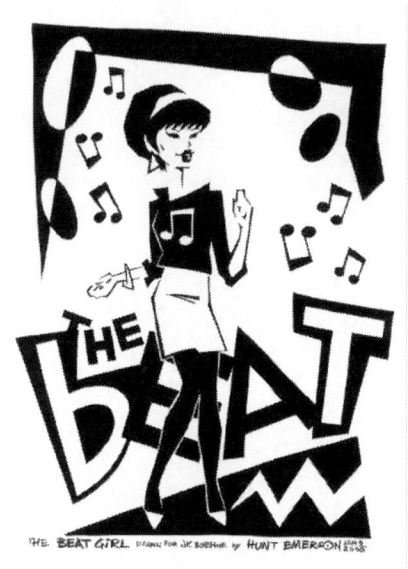

I went with my friends to see The Beat – the pop reggae band from the early 1980s (remember Mirror In the Bathroom?), who are still working, and are one of the best dance bands in the world. I designed their logos, record sleeves, and t-shirts, so obviously I have a certain preference... but we were all set for a great night out at Birmingham Town Hall. We got into the venue early and staked out a place we were going to be able to see the band without being right up front, and we chose well, because as the place filled up, our space seemed to be kept open.

The Beat came on, the place erupted, and we were having a great time. Then, a great lummox of a bloke staggered right in front of us. He was having a good time, but he was drunk and big. I wasn't having his, but I didn't want to push him away and ruin his evening and mine. So, I moved up to him and danced tai chi next to him. And of course, he found himself gently and mysteriously moved aside.

Just as he began to register that something was going on, I changed my balance and was no longer a threat to him, then when he was settled, I changed weight again, a sort of gentle "step up and play guitar" and he moved again… and so it went on, all in time to the bouncing ska/ reggae of The Beat. The guy was gently moved to another part of the floor, without even realizing it.

My friends, standing behind me, watched all this and said it was quite obvious to them what I was doing, and how the guy hadn't stood a chance – hadn't even realized there was a contest going on. Tai Chi principles of Softness proved themselves on that night.
Love and Peace, Bredren!

Rooting, Chi And The Mind.

The mind and the spirit must be strong in order to keep Chi from rising, which will destroy the effort of rooting.

The mind must be very centred and controlled.

Many people practice Chan (Zen) exercises, or something similar, in order to accomplish this. This, of course, has a parallel in life since the mind must also be kept centred every day in order to handle all circumstances that may occur.

When practising, one should use imagination so that one can imagine clouds or a river to create evenly flowing movement. One can go fast yet stay quiet.

When travelling in an airplane, one feels very still even though the speed may be 500 mph. Enemies to the mind are anger, fear, and various other emotions and distractions. They raise the tension in the body, making the muscles and joints tight and again can destroy the root.

All of these requirements to building root support each other and connect to each other in a complimentary fashion.

After a long time you will understand the harmony of the requirements.

The straight plumb line requirement causes the thigh to go in, but when one takes the two points in the hip out the knees move out opening the thighs up properly.

Another example of harmony between the requirements is that when the legs are down and when one sinks, the practitioner can use the whole body as a unit.

What kind of feeling is obtained from rooting? Should we feel something when we root?

The feeling that is derived from rooting is that the upper body is empty and the lower body is full. In push hands or in application where two people are linked together, if one person is rooting and the other is not, the lever principle comes into effect.

One person has the power of his chest and arms versus the other person using their entire body as a unit.

Everything else being equal, the unitary rooted person has three times the leverage. It is like someone who is standing on ice pushing hands with a person on dry ground.

Another feeling derived from rooting is that of smooth movement. The body turns as a unit; it also gives turning a greater range of motion. The body can turn in any direction.

Whether in fighting application or when interacting with a partner in push hands, one must yield and follow the opponent or the root can be shattered.

Root also allows the body to calm down and feel centred.

The principle of rooting is a product of the principle coming from the TAO TE CHING, the most famous book in China.

The Tao Teh Ching was written by Lao Tzu who described the way of the of the universe. This book told how to control the world. Its conclusion was that you control the world by controlling yourself; that you have more control in this world if you simply learn to control yourself and balance.

As this idea was factored into the internal martial art, it was discovered that when one learns to root, he has much greater control of his own balance as well as greater potential of power coming from the ground.

It is said Sun Lu Tang the famous internal martial artist who wrote Xing-Yi Quan Xue, (The Study of Form-Mind Boxing) did not think there was any secret way to practice the martial arts. He emphasized that there were two words which described correct practice, they where Zhong He, which translates to mean 'balanced' or 'neutral'.

It is always easier to reach a goal if the goal is very clear. Why be rooted in martial movement? It is because our goal is to be balanced. Rooting is most often compared to 'being like a tree' and so can be misinterpreted as strong and fixed but that is not what is meant. Rooting is 'neutral' and even Prof Cheng Man Ching is quoted as saying "rooting is natural, you just have to stop resisting gravity". Rooting is to achieve natural alignment, to be in neutral, with no resistance in an direction just alignment. Rooting enables natural compression to happen.

Stability

Jason Yeung likens the Tai Chi form sequence of *SEPARATE AND KICK WITH HEEL* as taking on the look of a circus high wire act!!! Balanced on one leg arms thrust out to the sides for stability he has a good point.

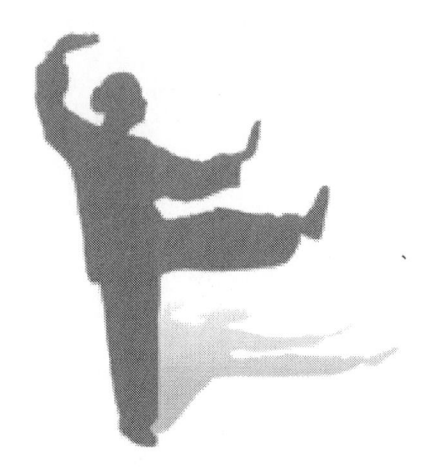

It is one of the most challenging moves you will encounter in the form.

It is just as challenging to the experienced student so beginners should take consolation from this.

Once you are accustomed to this sequence of moves it can be quite enjoyable to practice. Within it is a nice ebb and flow.

When feeling unsure or unfocused, you may start to wobble, become unbalanced, and occasionally calamity! You fall.

We know that the lower one's root, the more stable the posture. This move however, has three limbs making dramatic outward gestures, so it is logical that when that when coupled with the nervous anticipation that may accompany a difficult move such as this, your stability may be compromised.

So let's split this into several aspects:

PREPARATION: Is your body in proper alignment and stable from the previous move. Are your feet and joints flexible? Is the mind calm? Is the leg low enough to the ground that is does not disturb your balance too greatly.

LIFTING THE LEG: The weight must be settled deep into the root before lifting the empty leg outward. While the arms are used to counter balance the leg movement as it goes up and out. One must remember that moving the whole outward in this way transfers a great percentage of the body weight away from one's centre of gravity.
To this is added the momentum of the rising leg, also going out away from the body. It can be no surprise then that balance is challenged

BRINGING THE LEG IN: You must try and bring the leg in toward your root rather than let it drop back. Though gravity is the primary force at work as the leg comes back, if the focus is on the gravitational pull, it may create a bounce in the body. If however, you keep the focus on the root, the force will be transferred into the ground and you will remain more stable.

COMPLETION/TRANSACTION: If you feel a sense of relief on completion of the move you where probably anxious about it before you even started, aim for this relaxation before you begin the move. This move above all requires strict adherence to the Tai Chi principles. It is a great chance to hone your skills. Weather the leg is being lifted high or you are stepping out comfortably low, the only difference will be the mechanics and, most importantly, the mind-set.

Am I in a Tai Chi Trance?

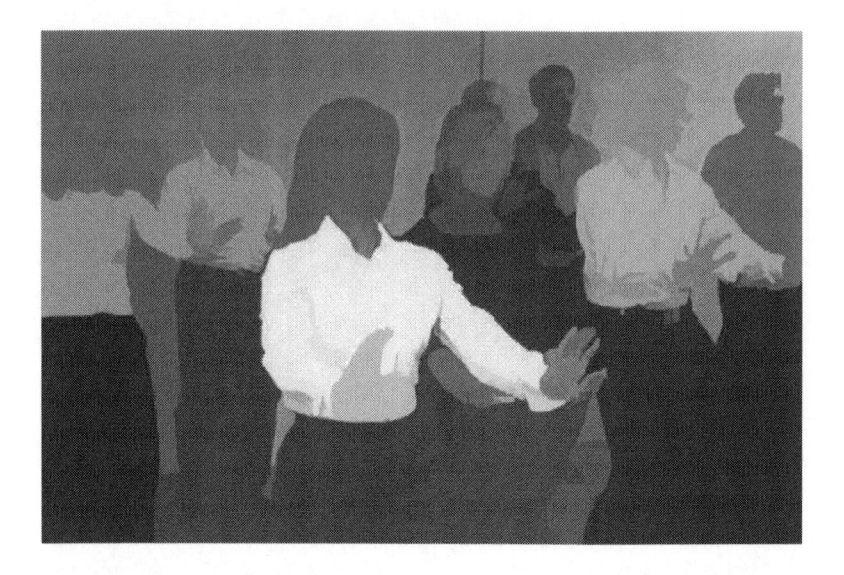

I was recently rereading a book entitled "My voice will go with you – Teaching tales of Milton Erickson". When I reached the chapter discussing research into autohypnosis (trances) in Balinese culture; it seems that the use of trance states is part of their culture even to the point where researchers discovered people would go into a deep trance on their way to the market and stay in a trance through the whole shopping experience. It struck a chord for me as I'm fascinated how trance states occur and are used especially if we consider a trance is not just some sort of stage hypnosis trick, but actually just a focused state of attention/intention. My old tai chi teacher Nigel Sutton often discussed the importance of Martial Spirit - having the correct state of mind (spirit) in training and application - as essential in proper development. A friend and exceptional martial artist, Chris Parker, talked about going into trance whilst he practiced Silat, and there are many more examples I could quote.

With the Balinese research they found that people would start with body-orientation movement that involved closing their hands, attempting to stand on tip-toes etc. to connect to the here and now through getting reacquainted with their body. The movements acted both as awareness exercise and as a trigger for the trance state they wanted to access. It is the same process that is used in mindful meditation and even chi-kung to create/access the relaxed state of awareness.

With all this in mind, am I in a tai chi trance and what does that mean? The first movement in the Cheng Man Ching form is 'Preparation' – preparing yourself and becoming body-orientated; from here we move into beginning. At first beginners are more focussed on just remembering the sequence but with practice preparation and beginning set the tone for the sequence to come and the intention set is played through; maybe you practice your form for balance, for flow, for spatial awareness, for connectedness, for martial application or any one of many possibilities and as you do the mindful attention is your developing tai chi trance. Maybe you use your imagination to play with 'what if' scenarios of defending against attackers or walking through an uneven terrain or working with the air around you as if you're swimming in it.

All of this mindful play is your tai chi trance development. What trance do you enter when practicing tai chi weapon forms? What trance do you enter when practicing sword-play? How about push-hands? A push-hands trance can enable you to give up to the flow of the interplay so as to enable your unconscious mind to learn and hone your body skills with your conscious fears and disbeliefs removed. Being in a trance does not mean not paying attention; have you ever considered your daily journey to work which follows virtually the same route every time and how you often don't even remember making that journey yet you still arrive safely as usual; if some part of you was not aware then how do you do it?

Some of you may be aware that I am trained in hypnotherapy, NLP and CBT. Through my training and experience I have found that its peoples conscious fears and beliefs, in the most, that cause them to have problems. In tai chi it is people's conscious limiting beliefs that prevent them from learning or progressing as their inner naysayer gets in the way. Yet when we change our focus of attention and develop the tai chi trance, it bypasses cognitive resistance and lets the inner explorer free.

Please practice to develop your tai chi trance and experience new levels of tai chi skill as you suspend conscious disbelief. Your unconscious mind already knows far more than you realise so set it free and enjoy your journey.

> *Fall down*
> *Seven times*
> *Get up eight*

Some Things Don't Change Or Do They?

When Mark first started teaching, and later when KAIMING was formed, we were always interested in why people became students of Tai chi, and had questionnaires that were on the back of the insurance forms that had to be completed and this 'why' question was asked amongst others.

Obviously back then as now the most recurrent replies where—— to help with anxiety, to be able to defend myself without aggression, always liked the 'look' of it, heard it might help with balance and was a gentle but healthy exercise.

When asked later when they had been students for a while, why they had continued after the first 10 week block of lessons and what their thoughts where now, a new reason had surfaced.

They found that because of the need for focus on movement and body alignment when learning the form (and later correcting detail after they had finished it), worries and stresses from work, problems at home, busy moms days, and general anxieties from life where all left behind for an hour when they practiced in the class, and they left feeling relaxed and fresh.

The warm up exercises loosened tense muscles in the neck, back, hips and legs; it gave people the chance to relax and have a friendly chat with the student next to them, and a feeling of camaraderie built up over the weeks.

When learning the postures audio, visual and kinaesthetic senses became acute and focus moved to each new area that was being worked on that week.

However this did not mean that there was no time to laugh with each other over attempts to master a difficult posture or even maybe feel a little glow of pride when the instructor passed by and congratulated you on "having got it". Even if you weren't sure what 'it' was!

Then as time passed and they began to feel more confident with their form and ability, and mastery of the art seemed to be on the horizon, suddenly a posture felt not quite right, or a knee or shoulder ached and that could mean only one thing, loss of focus and a little bit of complacency.

If you lose correct alignment your muscles and joints will let you know and you need to go back to the 'drawing board' or should I say basics.
I remember when I used to teach a class at the local gym a lot of the people who came to 'have a go' where more used to pumping up muscles than relaxing them off, so really did not move correctly when slowed down.

Their mind set was very different and because of this the movement of the skeleton on a different scale. They didn't sink the hips to turn, the neck turned independently of the rest of the body, and so did their knees very often.
After a session of showing them what they were doing wrong by demonstrating several movements a few times, I can remember the next day I had neck and knee ache, the class however reported back the week after a general improvement of their aches and pains!!!
If you ask me what I think has been the reason I kept on the Tai Chi path (apart from the fact I wouldn't have seen much of Mark if I hadn't) I would say two things really.
(1) I feel there is always something to learn or improve on, and sometimes as strange as it may seem it is a "new recruit" to the class who brings something to your attention with a simple question.
(20 The other reason is simply the fact I have learnt so much about my own 'body problems' after years of nursing, and how to find the answers to put them right that I am now in a much better place than I would be if Tai Chi had not been in my life.
I hope all our students and Instructors continue to enjoy their journey and find the commitment to continue reaping it's benefits.

Training Method For Tai Chi Chuan

Yang Ban Hou (1875), son of Yang Cheng Fu.

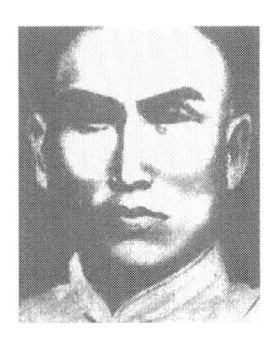

The eight trigrams and five elements are innate within us. You must first understand that they are based in these four terms: perception, realization, activation, action. [These four terms amount to "moving with awareness". Once you have achieved moving with awareness, then you will be able to identify energies.

Once you can identify energies, then you will be able to be miraculous (natural and free). But in the beginning of training, you should understand moving with awareness. Although it is innate, it is nevertheless hard to achieve within oneself.

In your own training of each posture, once you have learned them all, they are joined together to make a long routine, flowing on and on without interruption, one posture after another, and thus it is called Long Boxing. It is crucial for the set of postures to be performed consistently, otherwise it may after a while turn instead into either "slippery boxing" or "stiff boxing". You assuredly must not lose your pliability, and the movement of your whole body should be grounded upon mind and spirit. After practicing over a long period of time, you will naturally have a breakthrough and attain everything you have been working toward, and nothing will be strong enough to stand up against you.

When working with a partner, the four techniques of ward-off, rollback, press, and push are the first of the thirteen dynamics to work on. Stand in one place and do the four techniques rolling in circles, then do them advancing and retreating, doing them at a middle height. Then do them higher and lower as well, practicing at all three heights. Starting with the basics, work your way through the solo set. Then begin working with the four techniques, larger gross movements at first, then focusing on the finer details until the skill of extending and contracting is fluent, and you will have ascended through the midway of attainment, and then will continue to the top.

Work first at training gross movements, then finer details. When the gross movements are obtained, then the finer movements can be talked of. When the finer movements are obtained, then measures of a foot and below can be talked of. When your skill has progressed to the level of a foot, then you can progress to the level of an inch, then to a tenth of an inch, then to the width of a hair. This is what is meant by the principle of reducing measurements. Pay attention to detail but detail in stages.

Passing On The Art

Mr. Liu (Liu Shih-Hung) said that Professor Cheng once called for him to come over to his home. When he arrived, through the door he could see the Professor doing the exercise we know as "Constant Bear" (i.e., shifting and closing the kua on the loaded side with suspended head-top) as he worked with a manuscript. Professor continued the movement without speaking. Mr. Liu waited patiently and observed, feeling sure that Professor had noticed his arrival. Finally, Professor Cheng looked up at Mr. Liu and said, "This single movement is Tai Chi Chuan. Everything is contained in this." This exchange was the inspiration for Mr. Liu's basic exercises.

The "five animals" exercises grew out of Mr. Liu's meditations on some notes left by Professor Cheng (perhaps related to Hua To's ancient Five Animals exercise) and passed along after his death by Madame Cheng to Mr. Liu. The five are: dragon, tiger, bear, monkey, and bird. The nature of these movements (coiling/curved, pouncing/linear, etc.) correspond to certain postures (obviously we could describe differences in the movements and functions of the postures), but the principles are the same. "Return to the One."

For more info see Robert W. Smith's "Martial Musings" (he has a whole chapter on Mr. Liu), also Cheng Man-ching's "An Explanation of the Constant Bear" from master of 5 excellences

We listen to someone playing a piece of music composed by a great musician, maybe from long ago. We may have heard the same piece many times played by many different people, and what we hear is THEIR interpretation of the same melody.

Sometimes it may seem that it is totally different tune and that is because this is how the person performing it has changed or adjusted the basic notes to suit their style or maybe even find it easier for them to connect to the rhythm.

See the similarity with Tai Chi?

Masters have passed on the art over and over again down the years and their students have all received the foundations of what will eventually become THEIR interpretation of the same principles.

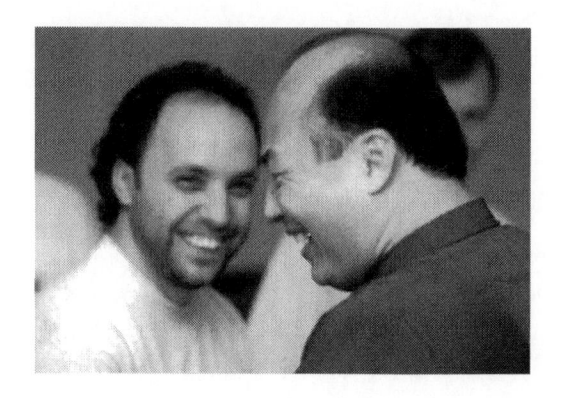

I asked MASTER TANG CHING NGEE of Singapore, when he was staying with us some years ago, "If someone because of some disability cannot perform some of the postures as they are taught, or maybe a posture in the form causes discomfort even practised correctly, will it affect the benefits they receive from Tai Chi?"

He replied that as long as the basic principles where followed and their body felt more comfortable with the posture performed to their limitations, or adaptations, it would make no difference. It is better to do what you can easily, than to feel stressed forcing a posture because you feel you have to.

Your instructor is there to help you interpret the music of Tai Chi......

The rhythm that flows through your body is yours!

Q&A On Tao Of Tai Chi Chuan. By Master Huang Sheng Shyan

There are different forms of Tai Chi. Are the principles different?
The founder created the art. But through the years, the forms of Tai Chi have differed:
some have 24 basic movements while others have 37; some have 64 set movements and some have 72 while others have 108 movements or even 124. There are long sets and short sets. Movements have been large and expansive and have been small and compact. Some emphasized high postures others opt for low ones. Some practice slowly others practice at a faster pace.

What is important is that the principles remain the same. Different masters with different temperament have been following the basic principles through the ages. They have engaged in continuous research and training. They have reviewed and improved the art until the ultimate objective is achieved where form becomes formless, limbs are no more important, brute force becomes non-existent and stiffness has given way to being fully relaxed. Character formation has advanced to the stage of "non-self" and of non-resistance so that the whole body is used and hands are no more used as hands. Youthfulness and longevity are attained.

It is not easy to master correct forms as the chi and the principles of the art are internally harmonized. Harmonization is also to be achieved between the upper, middle, and lower parts and between the left and right of the body. Even though difficult it is relatively easier to master correct forms compared to acquiring skill in the art.

This is so as in training or practicing there are a number of normally undetectable parts of the body that are difficult to keep under control from the aspects of speed, timing, rhythm, and balance. Because of this, skill in the art is difficult to acquire. But then as the founder says, "Understanding one portion of the art would mean being enlightened on all portions or parts. Then all schools and sects become one."

I like to think of this as what Willie Lim calls "the one elusive move". It doesn't matter how many moves, how many forms, how many patterns are practiced if they are not practiced with attention to detail and the guidelines laid down in the classics. I fell in love with Cheng's 37 step form and feel it is more than enough for a lifetimes study of enjoyment and refinement; each time I look outside of it to broaden my tai chi skills, I find myself lead back into it as all is there already. There are no secrets, there is only a requirement of an open and inquisitive mind to realize that the form is purely a vehicle to travel the tai chi journey in.

For what Purpose?

The aim of Kai Ming is to encourage and develop a love for the exploration and practice of Tai Chi Chuan as expounded by Cheng Man Ching. He strove for the essence of the art, not to mimic others; he practiced out of love, not ego. He encouraged the development of those around him without holding back.

With this in mind, I came across the quote below which I hope touch you as they did me.
Jenny Peters
"Even though our path is completely different from the warrior arts of the past, it is not necessary to abandon totally the old ways. Absorb venerable traditions into this new Art by clothing them with fresh garments, and build on the classic styles to create better forms".
(how good is that!)
Taken from THE ART OF PEACE

Part 6 – Martial Application

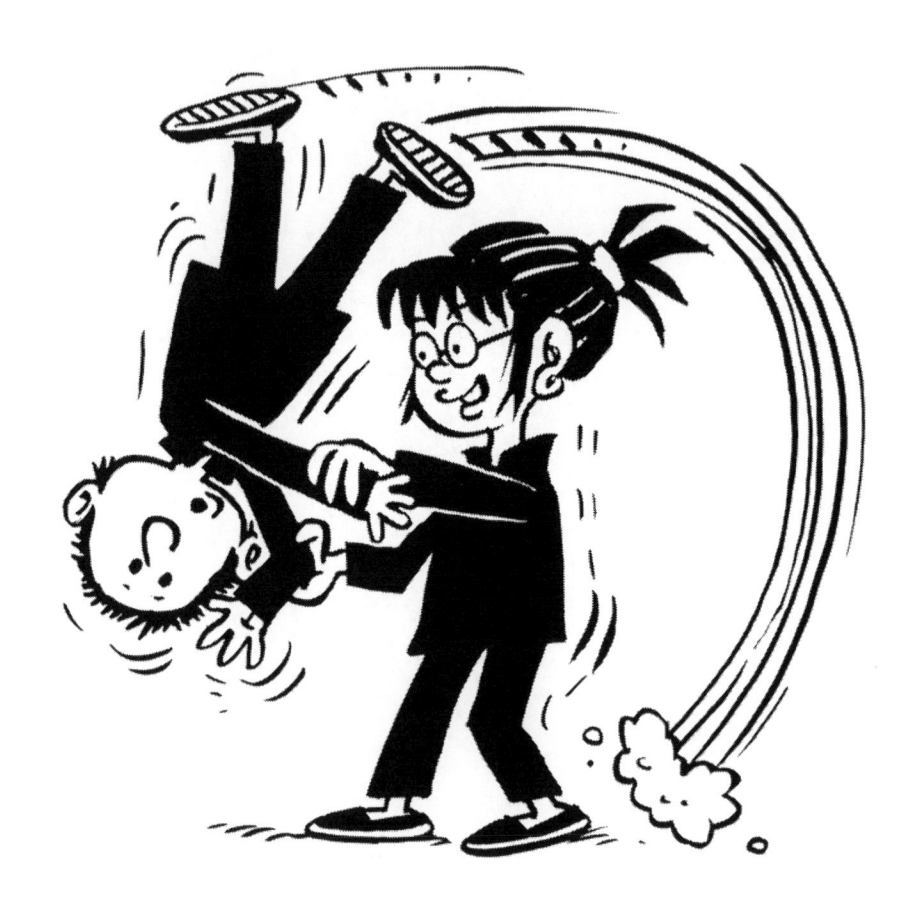

The Art Of Not Fighting?

A Tibetan Tai Chi practitioner who became engaged in a discussion of the martial arts and Buddhist doctrine, or dharma mentioned that although there are numerous references to the relationship between these two disciplines many generations after the inception of Buddhism, he could find nothing in the texts directly attributed to the Buddha on martial arts or attitudes.

His reply was that the martial arts are concerned with self-defence, and as there is NO SELF, according to the dharma, he wondered exactly what it was that I wanted to defend!

Although there is no mention of martial training in the sutras, there is an account of a confrontation that illustrates the desired attitude.

The Buddha, Shakyamuni, had a cousin, Devadatta, who was jealous of his success and popularity.

There are many accounts of his attempts to upset the emerging order of the monks and followers with varying degrees of success.

Eventually, feeling frustrated at his own lack of progress, he decided to murder his cousin and simply take over his position. To accomplish this, he strapped blades to the tusks of a rogue elephant and set him upon the path that Shakyamuni was taking.

As the story goes, the elephant began his charge, only to be totally subdued by the presence and non-aggressive demeanour of the Buddha, finally kneeling before him.

Religious stories do not exist as historical depictions of true events but as indicators of the correct behaviour and attitudes as professed by their creators.

Whether or not there is any conventional truth in this story, there are intrinsic truths that reveal traditional warrior values as developed in the East and even the highest approach to fighting, that of non-fighting.

The Buddha did not speak of martial skill, except as an example of mindfulness because he would not let a situation develop to the point or along the lines that lead to physical contact.

Fighting rarely, if ever, solves anything.

Only between honourable individuals could combat possibly resolve a dispute; but if both parties are honourable, where is the need to fight?

In Tai Chi Chuan, much is made of the accomplished practitioner who can receive full blows but remain unharmed.

This is attributed to the fact that they can stay very relaxed and open in the fearless knowledge that he can take enormous punishment if necessary, an important consideration in a culture where many of the fighting arts specifically develop bone-breaking and organ-rupturing techniques. Just take a look at this picture of Dan Docherty, a friend of Marks and highly respected tai chi master in the UK. This relaxation allows one to use Tai Chi most effectively and creatively.

Another story told is this—Yagyu Munenori, a Yagyu-Shrinkage school of swordsmanship headmaster and teacher of the shogun, was once approached by a young Tokugawa retainer with whom he was not familiar. Upon being questioned as to his identity by the sword master, the retainer replied that he had just been promoted to the palace guard and had been sent to hone his fighting skills.

He advised Munenori that he was not very good and that it would take a lot of work.

They crossed swords. Immediately Munenori the master lowered his sword and said there must be trust between a teacher and his pupil.

He told the pupil that although he had portrayed himself as a poor fighter, when they crossed blades he knew HE was facing a master.

Although the retainer insisted he was not lying Munenori asked him to tell him about himself and his training.

Born as a Samurai, the retainer said that it was his duty to carry a sword and learn how to use it.

Early on, however, he came to grips with the fact that he was not very good at it.

As it was likely that at some time he would be facing an opponent in mortal combat, he decided that it would be best if he could face death with a calm mind.

So rather than train at the sword, he spent many hours in contemplation of death.

As a result, he now had not the slightest fear and is ready to die.

Munenori smiled and replied that he had attained what their training is all about and presented him with a certificate of accomplishment!

The stories depict men whose pursuit of self-knowledge spilled over into the martial world.

The monk and the Buddha were seekers and not warriors at all, and the retainer was a poor swordsman using self-knowledge to ready himself for the inevitable.

As I mentioned above, the monk and the Buddha were seekers not fighters. But what of the many people who were not interested in enlightenment and wanted to become or improve as a fighter. The mental aspects of training have many benefits on all levels.

No-Self exists on different levels also. You do not have to attain the ultimate to profit from training along the way.

Links between the mind and breath will be noticed practising in meditation, yoga, tai chi or qigong.

The Tibetans say that "the mind rides upon the breath" (or loong, prana, chi) as a man rides upon a horse.

The Chinese say that were the mind is directed, the chi (qi) will follow. It also works the other way around. If one's chi is in the chest or shoulders, the result is physical tension and mental anxiety. Anger, depression, excitement, and joy all have accompanying changes in the rhythm of the breath and the placement of the chi. So does calmness, deep concentration, and enlightenment.

Just as entering meditation slows the breathing down this will lead one deeper into it.

Where the breath goes, the mind also follows. The aim of these disciplines is to make the mind take charge of the chi, rather than allow the chi to lead the mind around like a rider with a runaway horse.

Meeting aggression with aggression either verbal or physical is not a solution for anything, and you may end up feeling even worse about what has taken place or words that have been spoken that are un-retrievable.

Remember aggression and anger is also a form of communication for some. A fight is a relationship. Both have patterns of escalation. It may start with a tone in the voice, maybe the voice will raise, we stare, and maybe push, and then we fight, much as our primate relatives in the wild do.

However it takes "two to tango" and if you step out of the "dance" the aggressor is left confused and deflated.

By stepping aside (not taking the bait) you appear the superior combatant, you are showing calmness and the ability to think before you move, meanwhile they are powered by Adrenalin and even if they decide to continue the attack (physical or mental) you will have the upper hand and have time to gauge where the first "blow" will come from and how to parry it either with mind or body.

A CALM WARRIOR IS AN EXTREMELY DANGEROUS WARRIOR!

Jwang Dzu, the daoist sage, relates the story of a fighting cock. Briefly the cock was ready when it appeared to be made of wood, paying no attention to its opponents and thereby terrifying them.

There are no guarantees that you will always triumph. What is assured is that you will be as ready as possible for anything. One's integrity and spirit will never be compromised, especially when it is most important.

In the words of Carlos Castaneda, one is able to have a "gesture with death".

Like fighting with Taiji, which cannot be thought about or planned out, it must be spontaneous and totally part of one.

The calm is not something contrived. It must come from the gut and be a genuine expression of oneself; it cannot be manipulated.

It will only be attained by diligent practice of your Tai Chi, it will lead you into it naturally, and it will become one's unforced response to adversity.

The art of fighting without fighting is the highest attainment in any martial art, and surely this should be our aim.

Q&A From Huang Sheng-Shyan (Huang Xingxian)

Question: How should the movement be practiced in order they can be usefully applied?

Answer: Take the five loosening (or relaxing) exercises as an illustration. These exercises are based on Tai Chi principles. During practice there must be full concentration since any distraction will nullify any effects. Bear in mind the 3 points of non-mobility: the head which must be locked onto the body, the hands which must not move of its own volition and the soles of the feet which must be still and rooted to the ground. Consciousness (or intent) will lead the chi along. Steps are made without affecting or moving the body. Turning movements start from the waist and hips with hands propelled from the waist and hips in accordance with the principle that all movements originate from the waist. Principles must be understood and no movements are separated from the principles. Once you make it internally you are also 'through' externally.

Once you are fully relaxed, you can change according to circumstances and can therefore, neutralize an oncoming force. You would have reached that position of 'non-self' where the whole body is the weapon and hands are no more used as hands. If you are not able to usefully apply your movements then you still have not understood the basics of the five relaxing exercises. If you have not mastered the essentials, then there is no point of talking about application of the movements.

This week in class a long-standing student and Aikido instructor suddenly said *"Wow, I can see so many potential applications!"* this light-bulb moment happened when we were working on loosening the shoulder-blades and upper body in one of Huang's loosening exercises. We applied it to form movements and found that applications of strikes, locks, throws etc were generated not by the applicant but by the attackers energy; what I mean by this is they came out of the energy and direction of the attack rather than the defender looking for options. The non-self of just being and naturally responding felt like a free-flowing dance. For me, just being, stillness, mindfulness or whatever you want to call it is the true wonder of martial arts and in particular taijiquan (tai chi chuan).

Somebody said to me recently "I can't relax, sitting still and quiet just isn't me!" but they had missed the point, still and quiet are not a physical action alone they are a mental one. Stillness and quietness can and are found in movement. Stillness and quietness are the freedom between the movements, the quiet between the notes, the freedom of being in the here and now without being fettered by extraneous thoughts and feelings; as Deepak Chopra once said *"we are human beings not human doings."*

Even Prof. Cheng Said *"tai chi without function is no tai chi at all"* so why practice without application or attention? For me function isn't just fighting an opponent it's not fighting yourself…. Its application of mind and body… its being in the here and now in every instant and experiencing it as it happens… its applying my *ALL* to balance, space, time, flow etc etc etc….

How movements should be practiced in order they can be usefully applied? They should be practiced with full awareness and commitment!

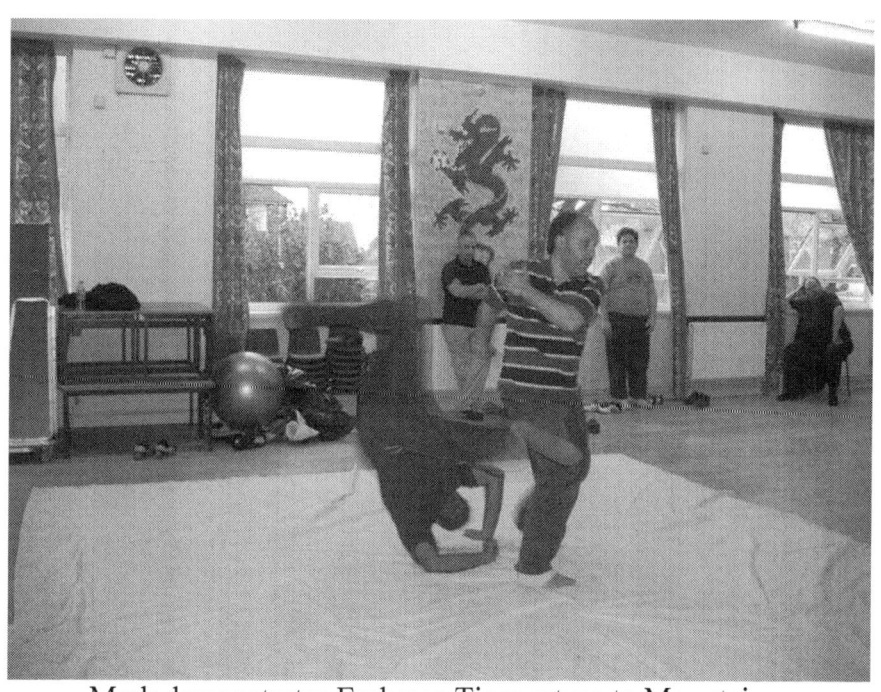

Mark demonstrates Embrace Tiger return to Mountain with Steve Fullerton

Tai Chi Chuan—Boxing for the Gentle

Robert Smith was beaten. The short, thin Chinese in his late 60s had let Robert punch him in the chest, abdomen and even the kidneys as hard as he could. The Chinese had only smiled and called for even harder blows, but Robert gave up. He had hurt his knuckles in trying too hard.

The old man smiled broadly, as he had so many times before. Robert smiled ruefully. It was his first time to be beaten by a man who had done virtually nothing to win.

Robert was not a weak man. In fact he was very strong. Back home in the States, he was a boxing coach. He learned judo in Japan, made the Third Order, Black Belt, and wrote a book about it. He was schooled in the Pai-kua, Shao-lin and Chin-na systems—the hard school of Chinese boxing that specifies force and violence. He weighed close to 200 pounds, mostly in bone and muscle.

But this old man was a Tai Chi Chuan practitioner who draws power and strength from deep abdominal breathing and bases his boxing skill on the principle of yielding. He had proved that force and drive are no match for ease and flexibility.

Accent on relaxation has made Tai Chi Chuan more than an art of self defence. It has become known as an excellent exercise for achieving mental relaxation through physical movement.

The power of nature is found in grace and ease, the Tai Chi Chuan exponents say. In Chinese, Tai Chi means "The Ultimate," the reason for all beings and the epitome of life.

A principle so complicated and yet so simple is not easy to conceptualize. It differs from what we are brought up to believe. Health and strength are not found in bulging biceps and hard muscles. A young lumberjack can be roundly defeated by an elderly scholar. To make the first move may be to lose the margin of victory.

All this has to be seen to be believed. Even then, it is easy to suspect that some malarky is involved.

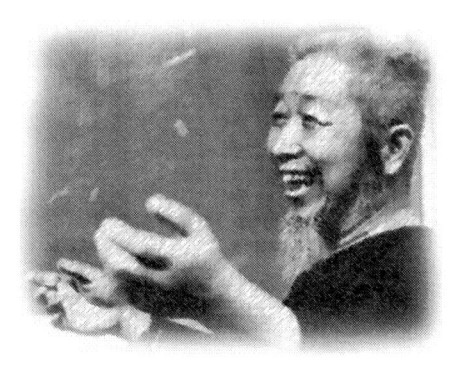

On **Taiwan Today**, the best man to disprove this is Prof. Cheng Man-ching, 61-year-old Chinese scholar who has been a master of Tai Chi Chuan for more than 30 years. He is one of the top disciples of Yang Cheng-fu, the reigning authority of his time.

The name of Yang Cheng-fu may not mean anything to those knowing nothing of Chinese boxing. But in the annals of the pugilism of China, he was among the most illustrious. His fistic feats have become legends. He was known to subdue his opponent even before he was even touched.

Chen Man-ching would not have learned the orthodox Tai Chi Chuan from Yang Cheng-fu had it not been for the revolution of 1911 that overthrew the Manchu Dynasty. Yang had been instructor in the imperial court, a most honoured post for any pugilist in those days. His teaching was monopolized by princes and members of royal families. Revolution made him jobless but it also gave him an opportunity to teach commoners. His fame spread far and wide.

Cheng at that time was a weak young man who had distinguished himself only in Chinese herb medicine practice. But he was suffering from T. B., which his herbs had failed to cure. He spat blood and had fever in the afternoon. Peptic disorders further enervated him. He was so weak that he could not sleep at night if he had walked more than a hundred paces during the day. He had almost given up his case as hopeless.

Yang Cheng-fu did not take a disciple easily. As a well-known doctor, Cheng one day was invited to treat Mrs. Yang, who was seriously ill. The diagnosis was brilliant and Mrs. Yang soon was well. Out of gratitude and impressed with Cheng's talent, Yang Cheng-fu taught Cheng the secrets of Tai Chi Chuan. It took seven years for Cheng to learn them all and go out on his own.

Cure Attested

In relating his past, Cheng never hesitates to reiterate his conviction that Tai Chi Chuan is a cure for T. B.

"My internal haemorrhages stopped and my temperature returned to normal within a few months of practice," he said. "In less than a year, my coughing was gone. But it took six or seven years to end headaches, loose teeth, dim eyesight and failure in concentration.

"I am now over 60 years old, and I can do everything anyone else is normally able to do. My eyesight is better than it was 30 years ago and I read small letters without the aid of glasses. My teeth are stronger than before."

Cheng's day is full of activities. A many-talented man, he divides his time among poetry, calligraphy, and Chinese painting in addition to herb medicine and Tai Chi Chuan. For years, he has been tutor of Chinese painting and calligraphy for Madame Chiang Kai-shek.

His is the story of rebirth. His primary purpose in learning Tai Chi Chuan was to improve his health. He said he never dreamed then that one day he would be able to beat nationally known pugilists.

Chinese pugilism is a tough and serious business. No hold or blow is barred or overruled. Boxers fight with fists, elbows, shoulders, knees, edges of the hands, fingers and feet — in ways designed to inflict different wounds on certain parts of the body. A Chinese pugilist gives no quarter and gets none.

In his career as Tai Chi Chuan authority, Cheng has been challenged many times. For years he was the director of the Pugilists' Association of Hunan Province. Hunan was the Mecca of Chinese pugilism. It was there that he met the toughest opponents of his life. Chinese boxers of all sorts came to test his mettle. They left with glowing respect.

Prof. Cheng doesn't close his doors to curious visitors, even now. Among them was a man called Liang, champion of the Shaolin School. Liang was a strapping man with, over-sized hands. He was ambitious. He had beaten too many to be modest. And now he must challenge Cheng Man-Ching to prove himself.

Through a common friend, Liang invited the old master to dinner. After a few drinks, he dropped his gauntlet. But Cheng Man-Ching smiled and said it was not his custom to show his boxing skills at a restaurant. Nevertheless, he would welcome Liang to have a "friendly bout" at his house.

The Challenger

At his unpretentious home, the master waited. Liang turned up on the second day. He was aggressive and refused to call it a day after he had lost in some minor contests. This taxed the patience of the master.

"Attack me any way you want," Prof. Cheng said. "If I am seen moving my hands in defence, call me a man without a family name." To lose one's family name is worse than death to an honourable Chinese. The witnesses were momentarily worried.

The Shaolin pugilist used the most deadly fist-and-leg onslaught. But at the point of contact, he bounced off as if he had been electrified. He crashed through a door yards away. No one on the scene saw Prof. Cheng move his hands.

The fall was not all. That night, Liang's head was swollen like a watermelon. As a boxer, he knew it was an inner wound and that no one except the man responsible could do anything about it. So he went back with humbled heart and Prof. Cheng gave him treatment. Liang wound up becoming a Tai Chi Chuan convert and began to take lessons from Prof. Cheng.

Eliminates ear

It is inconceivable to the uninitiated how a Tai Chi Chuan boxer trained only in physical and mental relaxation can fight a man of muscle. Relaxation is, in fact, the secret, and the degree of accomplishment is measured by one's ability to relax. The most advanced achieve a mental calm that is a great force in itself.

Prof. Cheng often says that Tai Chi Chuan is a mental process that eliminates fear, which is man's biggest enemy. Fear makes a man rigid, deprives him of flexibility and paralyzes both body and mind. When a student practices Tai Chi movements, he is taught to deal with an imaginary enemy who is strong and fierce. But when he is actually facing an opponent, he must imagine there is no one in front of him.

The appearance of Prof. Cheng as Tai Chi Chuan master is deceptive. He wears sideburns and whiskers. Chinese long gown and cloth-soled shoes are his everyday attire. On occasions, he puts on the gown-like dress he designed himself. He is more than unobtrusive; he looks sluggish.

That was the way he looked to me when I called upon him one autumn evening three years ago. He came to answer the door himself. His speech was relaxed and relaxing and he moved slowly. I wondered if I had made a mistake.

It was not until I had known Tai Chi Chuan for a year that I understood why the master walked the way he did. He was not walking, really. He was moving in the unhurried, continuous and relaxed way of Tai Chi Chuan, which had become a part of his living.

Footwork is of paramount importance to a Tai Chi Chuan practitioner. It is to his feet, or rather to his soles, that his weight and strength must go. From his soles spring his power and momentum. His push is designed to "uproot" his Opponent or to unbalance him so that he loses his mental equilibrium. But such "pushes" cannot be administered unless they come straight from the soles.

To be "pushed" by Prof. Cheng is unforgettable. I first had the experience in a friend's house where four Americans were also present. By way of explanation, Prof. Cheng asked me to stand about a foot and a half from the wall and place my hands on his arms to push him. I was no novice in Chinese boxing. I had devoted years in my school days to learning "crane boxing," and I had been pushed by strong men many times before in my life. But before I could exert pressure on his arms, I bounced off and hit the wall with a thud. It was a horrifying loss of balance. Failing to steady myself, I lurched to the right and smashed into a glass door three feet away. That was one of his gentlest pushes.

Now that I have studied Tai Chi Chuan for three years, I know it was not merely his strength that gave me such a strong push. It was my own force reflected on his sensitive hands. It was the desire to win and to muscle in quickly that undid me.

Ideal Exercise
Many Chinese learn Tai Chi Chuan for its health giving aspects. It is an exercise for all, young or old, male or female. Because of its complete emphasis on relaxation, it is almost effortless. Progress calls for more relaxation and concentration. Advanced Tai Chi pugilists learn to fill their "Tan Tien," the spot a little below the navel, with abdominal breathing. Prof. Chen says "Tan Tien" is the reservoir of vigour and vitality.

For one in search of an exercise that takes the minimum physical exertion but produces maximum effect, Tai Chi Chuan is ideal. I have watched men and women in their 60s take up the exercise with excellent results. After some time, they even managed to do such difficult movements as "the Snake Slips Downward", which calls for sitting on one foot in a squatting position while stretching out the other leg.

All Tai Chi Chuan movements have descriptive names. You have "Brush the Tail of Sparrow", "Golden Cock Stands on One Leg", "Embrace the Tiger to Return to the Mountain", "The Crane Spreads Its Wings" and many others. The set Cheng Man-ching learned from Yang Cheng-fu consisted of 128 movements. Prof. Cheng believed many of the repetitive movements could be cut out, so he spent years in shortening the set to 37 movements. His simplified version takes less than 10 minutes. To go through the movements both in the morning and before going to bed is more than enough to keep one fit and healthy.

Power of Passivity
The origin of Tai Chi Chuan dates to the time of Huang Ti, one of the earliest emperors of recorded Chinese history. It then was blended with the philosophy of Lao-tzu, who believed in the power of passivity. The movements of Tai Chi Chuan were not organized until toward the end of Sung Dynasty, some 800 years ago, when a Taoist leader named Chang San-feng devised the whole set.

The Taoists in those days spent most of their waking hours in contemplative sitting. Chang realized that lack of physical exercise might be harmful to health. Once he watched a snake fight a bird. The bird was jumping around and crying excitedly while the snake waited silently, its head poised for attack. The snake struck swiftly and surely and killed the bird instantly. Inspired by the ease of the snake's attack, Chang established the fundamental principle of Tai Chi Chuan that softness overcomes hardness.

Chang's disciples formed the school of Wutan Mountain. Temple feuds were common in those days and pugilism became an important institution among the monks. These were men without mundane cares who could afford to devote years to hard training and Spartan living to become good boxers. Rivalling the Wutan boxers of that time were the Buddhists at the Shaolin Temple, the seat of worshippers of brute force and physical impact. They were trained to split a stack of bricks with one blow of the hand and to send a man flying with a kick of the foot. A Shaolin trainee "graduated" by fighting his way through a tunnel equipped with boxing automatons.

Despite all the training of brawn, the Shaolin pugilists proved no match for the Wutan Tai Chi boxers. The vendetta has been a source of innumerable stories for China's writers on pugilism.

Like other arts and feats, Tai Chi Chuan has different sects. The school to which Prof. Cheng belongs is called Yang, the name of its founder.

Yang Lu-shan was a rich farmer in Hupei province in the middle of the Ching Dynasty, the last before the 1911 revolution. A man of good nature, he was constantly mauled and mistreated by local bullies. So he sought to defend himself by learning Tai Chi Chuan. He proved to be a genius and soon became the scourge of the bullies.

As the years passed, his fame spread. It reached such a peak that the court of the Ching Dynasty offered him the post of boxing dean at the royal palace. It meant he would be teaching members of the royal family exclusively, and so would be his sons and grandsons. The secrets were not to be handed down to daughters, in the tradition of the times, because they would not remain in the family.

Many Stories

The pugilistic feats of Yang Lu-shan made incredible stories but are alleged to have been true. Prince Dwan was sceptical. So in Yang's first evening at the imperial court, the young prince set loose two ferocious hounds. The dogs came at his legs but suddenly howled in retreat. Yang walked on as if nothing had happened. Next morning the dogs were found in their kennels, refusing to eat.

Other boxers at the court found their lucrative posts in jeopardy because of Yang's presence. They ganged up against him. One evening as Yang passed a deserted alley outside the court, more than a hundred embittered boxers attacked him with rods, stones and bricks. Yang squatted and covered his head with his hood, making no attempt to defend himself. To everyone present, he was beaten to a pulp. But he wasn't. The next morning he went about his business at the court as usual while those who beat him groaned in bed, their bodies bruised and painful.

Fantastic as the stories may seem, they aver the cardinal principle of Tai Chi Chuan: that force and violence used to hurt another hurts only the attacker. Tai Chi Chuan practitioners are so wary of the backfiring nature of force that they develop a touch so light and tentative it seems to come from a hand without bones.

All the movements of Tai Chi Chuan train the pupil to be as supple as a child. The hands of an accomplished Tai Chi boxer are usually fair-skinned and smooth. It is the "chi" that does it, Prof. Cheng would say. His hands are as fair as those of a maiden.

"Chi" is hard to explain. It is breath but it is not. It is blood circulation but not quite. It is mental concentration, perhaps. It could be an inner power moved by will. Nobody knows for sure. I am certain of only one thing. The more I know about Tai Chi Chuan, the less I care to subject it to scientific analysis.

No scientist himself, Prof. Cheng still has used physics to prove his points. He believes Tai Chi Chuan is one of China's greatest inventions and should be introduced to the West. During World War II, he staged two impressive demonstrations at the British Embassy and the American military mission in Chungking. In both cases, sturdy stalwarts experienced in Western boxing were selected to disprove his strength. None of their blows even landed. Instead of hitting him, they were sent lurching many feet away.

One towering giant of some 230 pounds tried twice. He was obviously perplexed by the inexplicable power of the small Chinese. Frustrated in the first attempt, he attacked even more violently. But force again undid him. He was tottering perilously toward a serious fall and the spectators were watching with apprehension. Before anyone knew what was happening Prof. Cheng had darted to his side to steady him with a soft hand on the elbow.

None would believe it as easily as Robert Smith. After studying Tai Chi Chuan under Prof. Cheng for almost two years, he still needs that tender and kindly hand to check his fall.

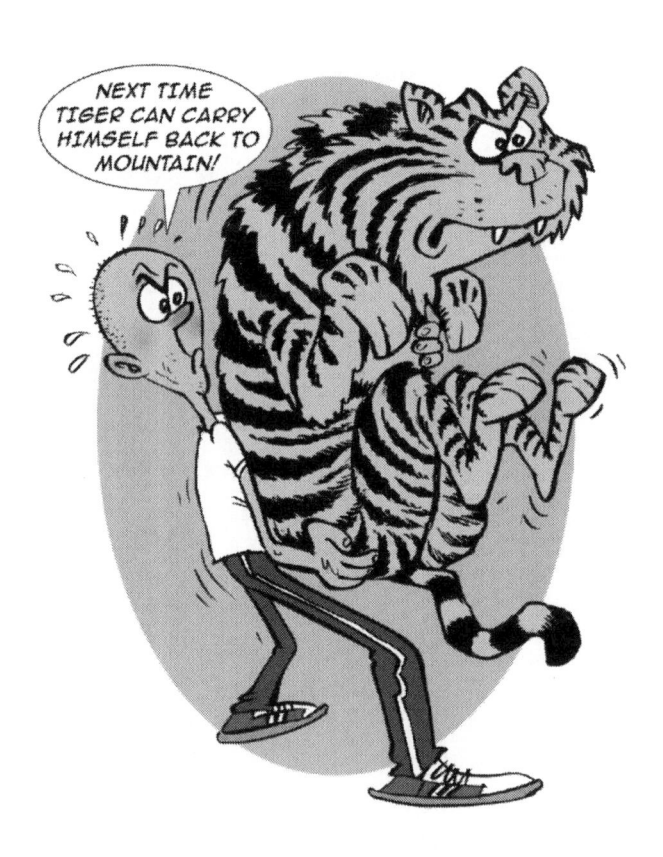

Training The Mind's Eye

The "mind's eye" is the way we perceive the outside world in relation to ourselves.

When you practice Tai Chi you may change the way others perceive "normal", by the way your practice develops.

By feeling the movement and practicing with intent and focus when performing the sets, we will all develop our own personal internal division of time based on the flow of the movement.

Eventually your movements can be much faster if needed, and you will still retain this internal division of time, because it was set previously at a slower pace and is "wired" in.

Movements performed quickly will still appear to have the slow-motion quality when seen through the internal "mind's eye" therefore you will function faster while retaining perception.

The brain receives messages very rapidly to perform physiological tasks, and equally sends messages back to create muscle movement from stimuli to our consciousness.

This is done so fast that the movement seems to be linked to the conscious thought e.g. reaching to pick something up, or open a door for instance, but the impulse was sent to and from the brain at the speed of light, so it appeared subconscious.

However in times of high anxiety, and other major distraction, the mind may become overwhelmed by the "noise" within.

The thought process may be scattered for a split second affecting our ability to perceive real time.

Martial artists must therefore realise the importance of developing a clear, calm mind.

Within our practice of Tai Chi we should always work towards calm, sinking, and relaxation to reduce tension and the discomfort that the fear of loss may bring. Only then will we see what is before us more clearly and be able to deal effectively with fearful situations, either physically or psychologically.

Elements Of Combatitive Tai Chi Chuan

Tai Chi initially became widely noted as a combat art when Yang Luchan bought it to Beijing where he taught at the imperial court.
Yang was challenged many times, but no one ever came even close to defeating him. His skill was so great that the martial artists bestowed on him the title "Yang the Invincible"
His grandson Yang Chengfu continued to promote the art until it spread far and wide. He taught his art in a combat style which also can be used to strengthen the body.
In his book THE PRACTICAL APPLICATION OF TAIJIQUAN he wrote—

In taijiquan, the ability to cultivate oneself physically and spiritually, but not to defend oneself, is civil accomplishment. The ability to defend oneself, but not to cultivate oneself, is martial accomplishment. The soft taiji method is the true taiji method. The ability to teach the art of self-cultivation and self-defence, both cultivation and application, is complete civil and martial taiji

Adapted from Douglas Wile's translation.

As we all know Taiji is very different from the hard-hitting, external martial forms. So what is combat taiji? It is not about great power even though it is capable of generating great power.
The Classics state clearly that the art is not based on great power.
Once when Yang Banhou had bested an opponent and was proud of himself because of it, Yang Luchan, his illustrious father, pointed to Banhou's torn sleeve and said that he was happy that Banhou had won but had he used taiji taiji to win? The implication is, of course, that a torn sleeve is a sign of inappropriately used power. Yang Luchan's own boxing was so soft that it was nicknamed "cotton fist" or "neutralizing fist."
It was once berated as not being combat effective because of its softness, a point which Yang refuted by promptly defeating the antagonizer!

The anatomical weapons in taiji are not rigorously hardened as in external styles of martial arts. This is because it is not hardness of the weapon but the energy within it that is the effecting component. If the correct structure of the anatomical weapon is maintained, then structurally it will be substantial and able to deliver telling blows with much power without recourse to hardening.

The appropriate and efficient use of strength usually does not require great excess to obtain the desired effect.

The principles behind the adage of "deflecting a thousand pounds with four ounces" hold true in taiji.

The aim of Taiji as a martial art is to stop violence conclusively without recourse to more violence.

Most of the time, violence is redirected against itself or rendered ineffectual. Hence, taiji practitioners usually overpower their opponents by just turning their own violence against themselves, educating them rather than hurting them. Violence begets violence. In taiji practice it is shown that violence acts against itself.

Can taiji therefore be used as an attacking art? It can, but violence should only be the last recourse, never the first.

Ego has no place in taiji as it gets in the way of efficient practice and usage of the art.

Taiji is an art to prolong life and health in peace and combat.

In its practice as combat, peace is learnt and cherished.

We learn the art in the hope that we never have to use it in a violent situation.

Our knowledge of violence and the consequences of it hopefully have made us choose to avoid the destructive paths in life.

Stillness In The Martial Arts

Movement and Stillness conspired one day...
In Chinese martial arts, stillness lies between each activity; like mortar to bricks, it binds together the actions of the artist. Like silence between notes of music, it renders the notes into melody.
Why stillness?
Ancient warfare and battles demanded unstinting activity, exhausting stamina. Fear, adrenaline, anger, panic — all mixed in hours and hours of clashing swords and skimming spears.
Then comes a lull in the barbarity; a moment of quiet in the middle of the melee; a "now" that might last an hour, a year —- or an instant.
The trained army knows how to regroup; the trained warrior does the same. His attention must immediately turn inward to recuperate and rejuvenate. Without some stillness, he might not be able to go on. Stillness unifies. The old saying goes:

"Movement on the outside; quiet within. Quiet on the outside; movement within."

Some martial skills are certainly based on movement. The most obvious are punching and kicking. Yet other skills grow out of stillness. Two examples are rooting and waiting (a sort of patience boxing), keeping control of oneself until the opponent makes his move.
The skill of rooting allows the practitioner to sink earthward until he seems to extend roots into the soil itself. One starts this type of training by simply standing and rooting. There are many other ways to gain leg strength, e.g., squats, running, weight lifting, but none of these methods gain rooting. If there were another way, the old masters would have discovered them.
Only when the great outer muscles fatigue and allow adjustment muscles to take over, only when the weight 'sinks' and ligaments and tendons are called upon to support the frame, do we enter the realm of strength that grows deep from inside and compounds with every minute of standing. Only under these conditions does strength internalise.

So strength and calm can be gained from stillness —— strength and calm, and something much more important for martial artists: self-knowledge.

There is probably no more intensely self-analytical exercise than that of quiet standing (Zhang Zhong). The muscles ache, the body craves movement; the mind is beset by a thousand wasps of thought. You itch, you remember a bill you forgot to pay, and you become angry. Slowly, all this dissolves into a world of attention that draws you into a universe of your own body and mind. After a while, you have to face the fact that it is the stillness itself you are fighting.

"Relax!" you say, over and over to your twin burdens of body and mind. Relax you do…. then you feel the ache in your hip or your tooth. Everything is trying to seduce you away from calmness.
You stick it out and happily the whole thing finally passes.

Later in the day you notice that something that bothered you previously no longer gets quite the same reaction from you. Maybe you feel calmer, maybe a little more open.
You can never be sure if the standing had anything to do with it, but the next day maybe you'll give it another try. Standing still, but searching for the stillness within you. It is hard to believe that you can take such a long journey without even moving.

There is a paradox in that we study combat in order to gain calmness.
So if you wish to learn calmness, you should practice calmness and stillness will come.

Tai Chi The Non-Discriminative Art

(or you don't have to be male to pack a punch)

"My painful knees have improved so much."
"The mobility in my aching neck is unbelievably better"
"I realised suddenly I wasn't using my inhaler as much"
"My stomach problems seem to have subsided"
"I can cope with the stress in my life now".

You'll probably be surprised to learn that these remarks all come from people practising a Martial Art, ***TAI CHI***

My husband chief instructor Mark Peters has always said, whether you come to the art to improve your health and reduce your stress levels, or to learn a practical martial art to protect yourself, you *"Buy one and get one free"* because you soon realise neither works without the other. It's such a subtle occurrence that often you don't even notice , then suddenly you're " The Peaceful Warrior".

The origins of the phase "The thinking man's martial art" may come from the same source as the inherit softness of Tai Chi's movements. Unlike many eternal or "hard" martial arts, that perhaps where developed by warriors or fighting men, I like to believe the theory that says Tai Chi practitioners way back where monks and scholars, men of peace who needed to defend themselves, but abhorred violence. They believed that the internal power the body can project, is far superior to muscular strength and less damaging to the health. These men had another thing in common, *patience*, unlike their western counterparts.

This is sad, because so many people are 'lost' to Tai Chi and it's benefits, either because it's not an instant health cure, or because the younger students lack the commitment that these days seems to exist only in Shaolin Temple's. Haven't they heard the phase "If it's worth having, it's worth waiting for", an old saying often proven true.

I had been a student of Tai Chi for a few years and recently realised when looking back over that time, what a long way, martial and health wise I have come. My life as a whole has become so much *wider*, and surely it's this width that's important, perhaps more than the length; this may be because my awareness in general has improved.

Students of Tai Chi are usually quite social people (and those who are not, very soon become so) I feel this is perhaps because they are looking for more than an hour or so instruction. Those who stay after the first few months seem to find the art becomes an integral part of everyday life. They train their body in the physical and the mind in the philosophical. To march up and down a training hall, and perform regimented external disciplines would not be enough for them. You need to *FEEL* Tai Chi, and as their training progresses, that's exactly what the dedicated student will achieve. Without wishing to appear over enthusiastic there have been times when even I have become almost evangelistic, when extolling its many virtues!

Women are very often in the minority in the field of Martial Arts. Those that do test the "water" are usually attracted to external disciplines, believing them to be the best option for their self-defence. They are mistaken. Be they black belt or not, when it comes to the crunch, if they are attacked, a strong member of the opposite sex would realistically triumph; this observation is by no way meant to appear derogatory to the art they practice. It is just a matter of body mechanics. Women's bodies in general are soft, sensitive and yielding, They are not naturally muscular and built to carry home the days hunting (only a couple of bags from Tesco's maybe) Yes they are mentally equal to their male counterpart, but it is physically unnatural for them to be as strong. I believe we are much better suited to the sensitive art of Tai Chi, where we can use our softness to our advantage, and make the odds more even.

Women do not have to try and rise to the man's strength, we can draw them into our softness and use the element of surprise to re-direct or take their balance. After all, do we women really want to appear hard and aggressive when there is no need, as you can achieve much more with a great deal less effort, and retain your femininity. As this extract from my Tai Chi Bible, "There are no secrets by Wolf Lowenthal" shows:

Here is where many women find difficulty. Professor Cheng said that women are naturally much more gifted in Tai Chi. Their understanding of sensitivity and softness usually takes men years to achieve. However, it can take a decade for their talent to "pay off". In the meantime, in an insensitive push hands environment, they will be shoved around and, probably most frustrating of all, be "taught" by stronger men who assume that because they are winning, they must know more.

Applying the virtues of softness is frustrating and difficult. All sincere push hands students (both men and women) must confront this problem. [page 33]

It becomes clear that to reap the health benefits from your practice of Tai Chi, relaxation and softness are essential, and this is the great gift we women can bring to the class. Over my years of training in push hands, many times women students have complained to me that they dislike pushing with their male counterparts because the man's ego sometimes gets in the way. It is very hard for a man to "Invest in loss", which is essential, but to invest in loss to a *woman* well I can see this must be doubly difficult. In most cases as soon as the woman gains some advantage and the male student starts to lose his balance (dare I say face) out comes 'brute force'. This may not be a problem for the woman who has learnt to harness her opponents strength, in fact the harder he becomes the easier it is to take him down; the stiff body is inflexible and unbalanced. However the newer lady practitioner who has not yet acquired understanding and skill to cope with the attack, may feel too threatened to want to continue.

Because of this we try not to include push hands into the class until at least 3 months into the course; people need to know each other and their teacher to feel comfortable. The awareness of each other's space allows us to build on this interaction, to the point where neither party worries about loss, and aggression pales into insignificance. How can either of you gain from an exercise fraught with tension; no health benefits would ever be achieved with a stiff, locked body.

It must be extremely difficult for external martial artists to understand why the Tai Chi Chuan student sees the art as a serious self-defence. It is not unknown for us to be the butt of the odd joke or two, as they watch the slow graceful movements. But when many of these external exponents can no longer practice their art due to damaged stiff joints and broken bones, they are surprised to find their Tai Chi counterpart can carry on and still be effect in later life if they wish. *A case of the tortoise beating the hare perhaps.*

One of the problems experienced in class can be that students cannot free spar, and therefore are unable to realistically test their ability as 'fighters'. Push hands will allow them to find spaces in their partners defences, improve sensitivity, and developed their root, but because the nature of the art is for powerful fast "take downs" of your attacker it would not be safe or practical to go further in a training situation.

We also sometimes forget that as your fellow student is practicing Tai Chi as well, there can be no real test of each other's ability, in the event of a real-life situation.

So how do we solve this problem? I personally practice any new techniques on my 6ft-4inch son, who luckily has no experience of Tai Chi. Due to my success in eluding his grabs, throttlings, and lunges and his frequent requests for a cold compress, we both have to accept that it does work . However as I improve and his bruising increases, he seems to have lost his enthusiasm, and I seem to have lost my fall guy "*Kateo*"

It is a sad fact, in this day and age, that we all need to be aware of the threat of violence, and the unprovoked attack that is especially relevant to women. Some may feel that training in a Martial Art discipline would provide them with confidence and peace of mind. Then why not choose one that's success does not depend on their strength, will hopefully improve their health, and last but not least, should keep stress levels down; the biggest killer of all.

I am a registered nurse and firmly believe that at least 50% of all the patients I see ,are suffering from stress related or provoked illnesses. Whether it be stomach ulcers, skin problems, heart disease, blood pressure, migraine, asthma or muscle spasm, the list could go on and on. Therefore I see no benefit from practicing an external martial art that works on the basis of stimulating the body to pump out adrenaline, which increases the heart rate, stiffens the muscles, quickens the respiration and prepares you for "fight or flight", which to my mind says Stress, Stress and more Stress. Surely we encounter enough of this in everyday life without deliberately setting out to invoke this response once or twice a week in class.

I realise that some people do enjoy the rigid training methods, and find that "hard" sessions seem to somehow release their stress and aggressions. Physically and mentally I tend to feel these people are the exception rather than the rule. In the long term their joints will remind them of their former training days.

As the founder of our style of Tai Chi, Professor Cheng Man Ching so eloquently put it, when asked by a student "Why learn Tai Chi", he replied "When you get to the point in your life when you know what you want, you'll have the strength to enjoy it". Who are we to argue with this!.

Putting The "Chuan" Back In Tai Chi Chuan

(OR Who Stole the Kidney?)

Whilst watching a class of Cheng style Tai Chi students practicing applications from the form I was amazed at how my former observations were re-enforced. Those who joined the club solely for relaxation and the arts health benefits were the ones who were enjoying the martial applications the most. Why is this, have they suddenly developed an aggressive streak; or is it, as I think, that whilst training with others in class, they have come to realise the principles of Tai Chi really work! What I mean by this, is that the self-defence aspects are accessible to most people regardless of age, sex or brawn. Unlike many external martial arts, Tai Chi, if taught correctly by a reputable teacher, will not cause joint damage or broken bones and can even alleviate existing injuries. Due to its non competitive nature, the ever present ego can also stay intact. The practice of push hands is based around the golden rule of *invest in loss* and therefore even if you do decide to enter a competition, and don't win the gold medal, but take back the learned experience, are you not still a winner?

There should be no pressure put on you to perform forms (katas) etc. in front of the class, and no rainbow of belts to work your way through. If you decide to become a teacher yourself, with the permission of your own instructor, then that's a different matter and entirely of your own choice. This concept makes Tai Chi a very social thing where students help one another and pass on their own personal pearls of wisdom. There is no rush, learn at your own pace and enjoy the experience.

Having said that, make no mistake, Tai Chi is not being taught properly, if it is not being taught as a complete art, both martial and meditative. There are self proclaimed Sifu's who devalue the martial aspect and promote it purely as a healthy exercise. Could this be because stress relief and health promotion can be very profitable? Don't get me wrong, I am not opposed to this area of Tai Chi but if it is to be passed on in such a clipped fashion will this not eventually cause it in its entirety to be lost? To truly teach and practice this art it must embody Yin and Yang, soft and hard; to teach one without the other is like having steak and kidney pie without the kidneys. Why call it Tai Chi Chuan (supreme ultimate fist) why not call it Qigong (breath exercise). A martial understanding is necessary to understand correct posture; you are being robbed, if you paid for a whole pie and only got half, wouldn't you demand a refund? Bear in mind you need the relaxation/meditation to develop internal power which in turn strengthens your health and fighting skills (you need to master the fighting skills to stop people laughing at you when you're moving so slowly!!).

I myself looked at Karate, Aikido and Wing Chun, and yes all of them had something to offer. Unfortunately when push came to shove (no pun intended), if my opponent was bigger and stronger than me, in a true attack I felt I'd lose. Tai Chi Chuan was the one that gave me the confidence to believe, if I used the principles correctly and developed my natural sensitivity, I would at least stand a chance. I felt I could avoid serious injury and equal if not overpower my seemingly stronger attacker. This is what any martial arts self-defence aspect is all about, having faith that it will work for you.

At a recent seminar, held by Master Nigel Sutton, on Tai Chi Chuan for self-defence, the first portion wasn't spent learning techniques as you might expect, but working on the mind. We discussed and practiced relaxation, meditation and the mental attitude necessary to develop the required state of mind.

The mental aspect of self-defence is initially the most important. Research over the last few years, in the criminal assault area, has shown time and time again that the person attacked usually has a "victims" demeanour and body language. I think we all have this within us - luckily, the majority of us keep it there, and outwardly remain confident when out and about in this increasingly violent world. This does not mean we swagger around the streets or a night-club for that matter, with the words "fancy your chance mate" emblazed on our chest, in fact, the majority of people never think about the danger they may be in but they are sub-consciously alert and keep good eye contact with anyone within their range; this is their first line of protection, and as a general rule, they do not attract the unwanted attention of a would-be attacker.

The victim's body language in contrast, exudes nervousness, with low eye contact, unease and poor posture, all highlighting his or her vulnerability to the trained criminal element "the easy mark".
Your first and most important self-defence, is your mental attitude - the ability to stay relaxed mentally and physically is the basis of most martial art and definitely Tai Chi. The problem for Westerners is that Tai Chi Chuan is not an ***instant Self Defence System***, it takes years for most students to attain the level of relaxation needed to adequately defend themselves. So, in this day and age of action movies and flash external martial arts Tai Chi has largely lost its ***Chuan*** and become widely practiced as the slow Chinese callisthenic exercise that gets constant media attention.

If that's all people want, fair enough, but why not try Yoga; do they really not want the whole art or are they just unaware of its existence. If you only learnt half the alphabet at school, what happens when you need to use all the letters? It's really quiet similar to just practicing Tai Chi for health and relaxation. I think this is what most serious students find out during the first few months of their course and then come to realise they want more. Some have tried other external arts and because of injury or permanent damage to joints cannot practice them any longer. They come to my husband's classes and are encouraged to find they can continue with a martial art as soft and yielding as Tai Chi. The mechanics of the art alone are usually enough to ease the injury.

Every student of Tai Chi Chuan should be offered the chance to learn the whole. Their teacher gives them an instrument whether the student plays heavy rock or a lullaby is their choice, but at least they should know there is a choice.

It never ceases to amaze me when people phone, inquiring about lessons, the high percentage that know absolutely nothing about the art. It's perfectly understandable that little is known about the martial aspect for unless you read the martial art periodicals, the only exposure it attracts on TV and your local press, is its supposed health improving properties. It is constantly left to the minority to wave the banner.

In my opinion, the first point we should all start at, before even searching out a reputable teacher, is **read a good book**; we are all influenced by our first impression. I myself began the quest for *enlightenment* after constantly seeing the words Tai Chi crop up in night school brochures (I hasten to add, this is not the best place to begin your classes, most students you meet there will have taken cookery the preceding term and probably flower arranging the next, not really the stuff serious quests are made of!!) I booked out **Tai Chi by Danny Conner** from the local library, sat on my patio on a lovely summers evening and read the whole book, unable to put it down. I turned to my husband (who at that time, after trying Kung Fu, Aikido etc., was still martially unfulfilled) and told him to read it also. An hour later he turned to me and said, "This is the one for me". Thank goodness we chose the right book the first time or our Tai Chi trail could have been vastly different. Even then it took about six months of searching to find a teacher who fulfilled the criteria he was looking for. We were lucky, we knew at the beginning there was a whole pie to be found.

The most informative easy read, for a complete novice, I have come across is ***An Introduction to Tai Chi by Alan Peck***. It gives a brief overview of different styles of the art as well as a list of recommended instructors (of which I am glad to say my husband is one). From there it is a steady climb up the ever increasing pile of hundreds of available titles; my personal favourites are ***There Are No Secrets by Wolfe Lowenthal*** and ***Tai Chi Supreme Ultimate by Lawrence Galante***. Steer clear of any books stating that theirs is the only true style or that drift off into the obscure (I'd be more specific but for fear of reprisals). My husband can get most titles and if not, he can recommend other sources.

The next stage is the teacher. The British Council For Chinese Martial Arts (BCCMA) and the Tai Chi Union for Great Britain (TCUGB) hold registers for reputable instructors.

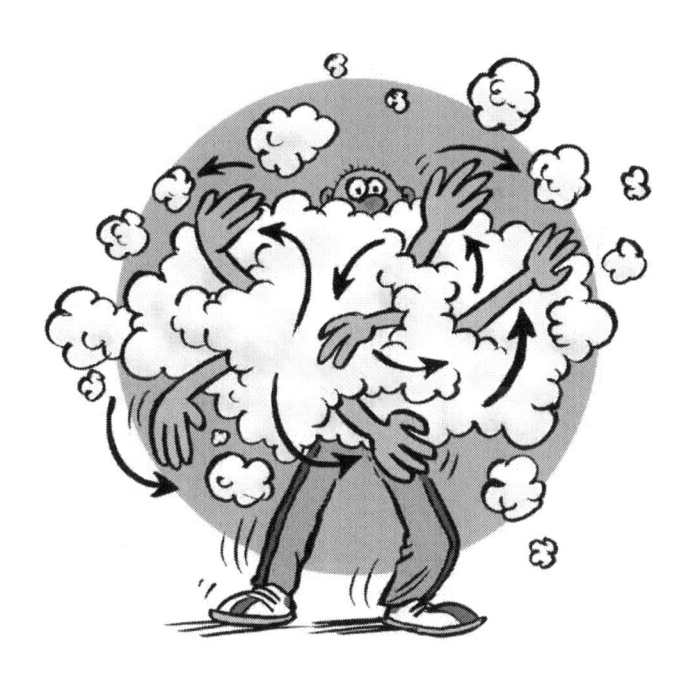

The Dying Art of "Stillness"

There are certain human changes which come about by participation in martial activities. The misunderstanding arises from the interpretive and market-oriented selling of martial arts to non-Asian communities.

It is hardly surprising in essentially a cultural marketplace that there exist newer, more generically made forms of martial arts (e.g. taekwondo, kickboxing, contemporary wushu), which are stripped of certain cultural nuances.

These absolutely fundamental aspects of the intent of these martial arts are continually underplayed as being culturally controversial, ethnographically unquantifiable, or simply incomprehensible to the observers. One of the more elusive cultural aspects is the relationship of the practitioner to STILLNESS.

In its original setting, stillness is considered to be a resource as well as an element of belief. Stillness and its direct perception are at the core of martial training. In Asian thought, this highly expedient method allows the practitioner direct access to models of experience with definite benefits.

One method is exemplified in stance training (Zhan zhuang) which refines the martial artist's skills with subtle, non-intrusive and profound re-association with his own body and mental processes. The constant attempt to strengthen and yet simultaneously relax (sung) offers an alternative to high level exercise which, though improving muscles, creates an aversion reaction in the body.

Stillness training circumvents this lactic-acid, adrenal-pumping approach and, in some instances, actualizes a more complete change in the body. At the same time, it establishes what, for want of a better term, we might call a 'default' system.

Just as the shoulder width stance is the natural First Position for the ballet dancer the horse stance or some variation of it (Wu Wei) must become the natural default position for a martial practitioner. The same process encourages a relaxed state of mind. Stripped of the normal amounts of fear and anticipation, this is considered the traditional default position for the practitioner's mind as well as body.

The obvious advantages in terms of increased reactive speed and clear judgments need not to be argued here. The point is that this training is the express agenda of the stillness practice, not a meaningless adjunct to it.

Even more profoundly, the concept that stillness is the "origin of all things" and that the practitioner must attach himself to it and learn from it, is an absolute requirement of Chinese martial arts. IT IS NOT AN OPTION.

This direct perceptual engagement is at the heart of the practice. Giving it up would be like attempting to teach science without referring to the cultural, objective, comprehensive materialism that is at the core of the discipline. In the study of physics, a basic and non-refutable core concept lies in the absolute similarity of quantifiable measurements and laws regardless of location (given the exigencies of local space and time conditions).

We find the same non-changing, unalterable premise in the twin concepts of selfhood and stillness. The direct perception of the Dao, individuated in the unique existence of the practitioner, is a fundamental proposition of the martial arts; it counterbalances the activity of the more frenetic aspects of the arts. It "rounds the corners" of practice. It re-associates the practitioner with the "original self".

The Original Self is a pressing consideration of Asian cultural modes. The very concept of self-defence is linked by definition to some comprehensive understanding of the "self" that is defended.

As mentioned in Sun Zi's The Art Of War, the overriding strategy here is "Know yourself and know your enemy and you will never meet defeat".

When practicing your form you look for stillness in movement, when practicing push-hands look for stillness in blending (connection to the other person). For me stillness in application is the difference between reacting and responding.

Part 7 – Epilogue – Beyond Tai Chi

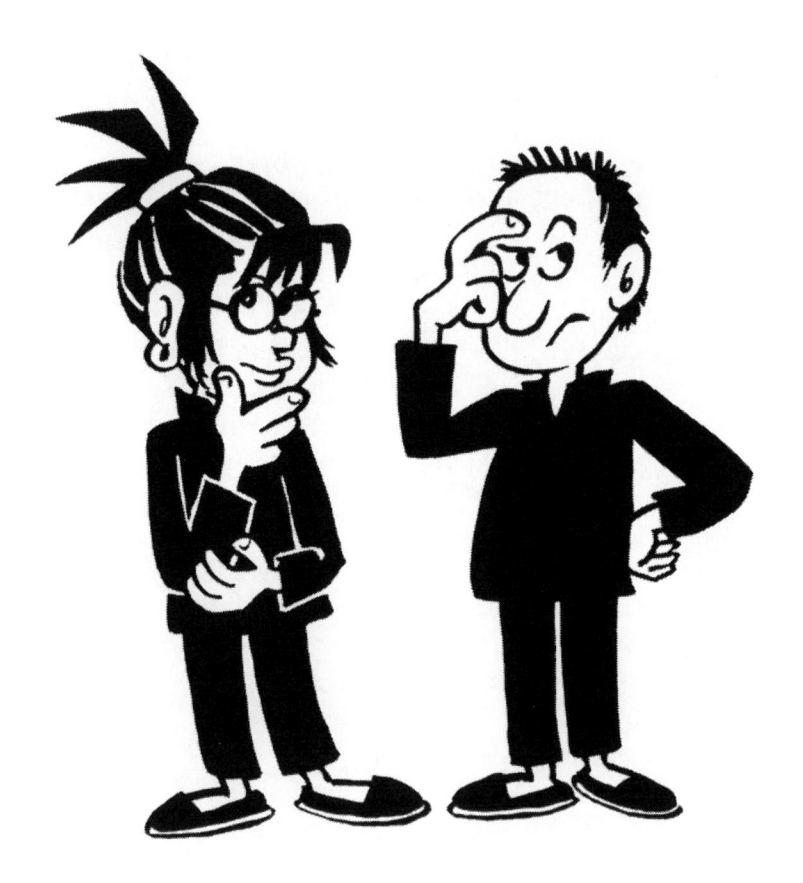

Thought For The Day...

I know the thought for the day is usually a Chinese quote (and don't they go on, how many ways can you say be an honourable person and live a good life!!). Well here's my interpretation of how we can do just that, in a few lines...

On Christmas eve I went to midnight mass, at a little church just outside Catshill, Worcestershire. Everyone who knows me will tell you I'm not overtly Christian but Christmas time is different, it has its own special memories for all of us, good and bad. For me it is a peaceful, special and almost magical time. We stood up with the congregation to sing "It comes upon the midnight clear"; I must have sung this hymn a hundred times during my life, and like many never really took notice of the words. This time, suddenly as I came to the last verse 2 lines stood out, why I don't know, but they seemed to make sense of many of the world's problems and what we need to do. These are the lines, interpret them how you will but do think about them....

Oh hush the noise, you men of strife, and hear the Angels sing.......

A story for Christmas..

By Colonel John Mansur
Taken from the reader's digest

Whatever their planned target, the mortar rounds landed in an orphanage run by a missionary group in the small Vietnamese village. The missionaries and one or two children were killed outright, and several more children were wounded, including one young girl about 8 years old. People from the village asked for medical help from a neighbouring town that had radio contact with the American forces. Finally, a US doctor and nurse arrived with only their medical kits. They established the girl was the most critically injured. Without quick action, she would die of shock and loss of blood. A transfusion was imperative, and a donor with a matching blood type was required. A quick test showed that neither American had the correct type, but several of the uninjured orphans did. The doctors spoke some pigeon Vietnamese and the nurse a smattering of French,. Using that
combination, together with much impromptu sign language, they tried to explain to their young, frightened
audience that unless they could replace some of the girls lost blood, she would certainly die. Then they asked if anyone would be willing to give blood. The request was met with wide-eyed silence. After several long moments, a small hand rose slowly and waveringly went up, dropped back down, and then went up
again. "Oh thank you", the nurse said in French, "what is your name?" "Heng", came the reply. Heng was
quickly laid on a pallet, his arm swabbed with alcohol, and a needle inserted in his vein. Through this ordeal Heng lay stiff and silent. After a moment, he let out a shuddering sob, quickly covering his face with his free hand. "is it hurting, Heng?" the doctor asked. Heng shook his head, but after a few moments another sob escaped, and once more he tried to cover up his crying. Again the doctor asked him if the needle hurt and again
Heng shook his head. But now his occasional sobs gave way to a steady, silent crying, his eyes screwed tightly
shut, his fist in his mouth to stifle his sobs. The medical team became concerned. Something was obviously

very wrong. At this point, a Vietnamese nurse arrived to help. Seeing the little ones distress, she spoke to him rapidly in Vietnamese listened to his reply and answered him in a soothing voice. After a moment, the patient stopped crying and looked questioning at the Vietnamese nurse. When she nodded, a look of great relief spread over his face. Glancing up, the nurse said quietly to the Americans, "he thought he was dying. He misunderstood you. He thought you had asked him to give all his blood so the little girl could live". "but why would he be willing to do that?" asked the navy nurse. The Vietnamese nurse repeated the question to the little boy, who answered simply, "she's my friend" Greater love hath no man than this, that he would lay down his life for his friends.

A Pause For Thought

If you can afford to cut back on work or overtime DO IT. go out with your partner or family and spend some quality time with them instead of worrying about what you could be catching up on! Or the extra money you are making.

If you cannot manage to have less income, think about what you spend money on that maybe you don't really need.

Do as we did, sit down work out the least amount of money per month you need to pay bills etc and still have treats occasionally (it will not hurt to not buy more games for the WII !) and then plan your work schedule around that figure.
If you can retire early DO IT! Especially if you will be under lots of stress by continuing to the Government's desired age, or at best cut down a couple of days in readiness.

You will not be bored, I guarantee it, and there are ssooooooo many things to do that far exceed the rewards? work gives us.

Just think, if you really get fed up you could go over Niagara Falls in a BARREL! Or not!!! Just a suggestion.
We all have dreams, try and make them reality, and don't always blame money for not attaining them.

"LIFE IS NOT MEASURED BY THE NUMBER OF BREATHS WE TAKE, BUT THE MOMENTS THAT TAKE OUR BREATH AWAY".

Chi, the Universe and Nan's Voodoo Wart Cure

When I was a small boy with freckles and ginger hair I had a lovely nan who could perform miracles. I first became aware of her magic when my cousin Lesley had a wart on her finger. OTC remedies and visits to the doctor worked for a short time but the wart would always come back, so nan decided to reveal her powers.

First she gathered the necessary materials: some bacon, a sharp knife and small cotton bag. Then, she put on her 'spirit travel scarf', and went into a 'trance', her eyes rolling back into her head just like Derek Accorah when Sam's not talking to him. She then mumbled to herself and cut the bacon so a piece fitted over the wart, mumbled some more and waved her hands theatrically over the bacon. Then with the obvious effort of keeping the warts essence locked in the bacon she lifted it off my cousin's hand and placed it in the bag. Lesley and I were completely under her spell and I had goose bumps as I felt the spirits gathering in the room. Then forbidding us to follow, "lest we become drawn to the spirit world", she went to the bottom of the garden, buried the bag and did a sort of dance over the "wart grave".

It came as no surprise to any of us when 3 days later Lesley's wart dropped off: it never came back. Word got around of Nan's powers and pretty soon everyone with a wart or bad spots or a sty would come to her. My nan would often joke about her skin colour (she was very dark) and claim that she must have African blood and when an uncle did a family tree and her heritage did happen to include an Afro Caribbean granddad, her powers became even better known and people would speculate that they were voodoo in origin. Only very quietly, as people were more than a little scared.

Nan's origins had another interesting affect. She had always been inordinately proud of her Celtic background and I think she truly ascribed her seemingly endless good luck to this.

Having found out that she was also part African nan became insufferable, and decided that along with her good luck, blarney and literary talents she now had a fantastic sense of rhythm and was a natural athlete. I think she felt she was some sort of hybrid of Oscar Wilde and Mohamed Ali.

Fast forward 15 years and I was staying with Nan during summer holiday, while at university. One night while watching spaghetti western (my Nan had a crush on Clint Eastwood) I asked her about her 'powers'. Nan became very still, drew in a breath and her eyes began to role. I felt goose bumps all over my body and waited in awe for whatever secret phantom she was about to reveal. Then nan sneezed and said "Don't be stupid Rob – I made it all up"

This made an impression upon me and over time I realised that a crucial part of some medicines is belief, and that belief is dependent on a good story. What constitutes a good story? In the case above, spirits, heritage, magic, the possibility of unseen power and the ability to control it. But good stories can be based on anything as long as they hang together and suspend disbelief. Take chi, meridians; exotic foreign concepts such as five elements and you have the base of a good story. Reinforce the belief by using needles to touch the body in places that produce minor changes that amplify that belief, and you have something quite powerful - in this case acupuncture.

So if belief is so powerful can we believe away cancer, believe ourselves young or fly? Maybe we can but we don't exist in isolation and we have lots of other believers super-imposing their beliefs. So while I may believe I can fly lots of other people don't, and more importantly, a flying human does not fit the known laws of science. One element of string theory suggests that the cosmos is no more than information – or maybe mind – so perhaps the laws of the universe exists because the universe believes they do? In other words no matter how much faith you have, you won't be able to fly until you come up with a way that complies with scientific laws, and perhaps those laws are the things the cosmos sees as following the plot - e.g. an aeroplane?

Now don't worry, I haven't lost my marbles, I don't claim that any of this is true and I have no evidence beyond conjecture. I am certainly not going to make the classic new-age mistake of wheeling out "post Newtonian physics" pretending that I understand it and using it as a panacea to back up anything I like, or claiming that sub atomic physics was invented by new age wizards.

Take the Taoist philosophy of tai chi often cited as some sort of ancient insight into the sub atomic world. The theory states that all things exist in a state of creative tension between opposites and this seems pretty true and to exist at all levels - even the sub atomic if you look at work on electrons as particles and waves.

However, the difference between the Taoists and Newton is that he didn't just notice, he produced tons of maths and theory around gravity: theory that is useful and repeatable and resulted in aeroplanes, suspension bridges and satellites. The Taoists noticed and then went off on a tangent about conserving you jing etc etc....

So is Western medicine a good story? In a way yes – the difference is that if you have an infection and you take antibiotics, no matter if you like the story or not, you are likely to get better. I think the universe likes the stories of antibiotics, surgery and chemotherapy: but it's not so sure on acupuncture or reiki, their plots seem full of holes. However, it did seem quite keen on Nan's voodoo wart cure.
By Rob Charteris – tai chi convert, Warwick

How To Please A Monkey!

The keeper said the monkeys were to have one banana in the morning and two at night.
The monkeys were very unhappy with this arrangement.

So the keeper said they could have two bananas in the morning and one at night.
The monkeys were very pleased with this arrangement.

The amount of 'bananas' remained the same; the secret was the adaptation to the likes and dislikes of those concerned.
CHUANG TZU - Wisdom from the East

Jenny read this saying to me because I'm constantly harping-on about NLP (neuro-linguistic programming) and hypnosis in respect to behavioural change; it made me realise its not about change but about change of perspective. We even had a new student come along to John & Lynne's class in Tamworth and say to me afterwards "I thought there would be more on breathing". Everyone comes with their point of view and our job is not to tell them its wrong but to understand how they have formed it so we can adapt to their expectations and then lead them into a wider understanding of this wondrous art we call tai chi chuan. It (Tai Chi) is no more difficult than anything else is to learn and its potential benefits are boundless from martial arts self-defence to a sort of self-defence against the stresses and strains of daily life. The skilfulness of a good teacher is found in adaptability; and here is a chance for me to quote an NLP presupposition, **"there are no difficult students just inflexible tutors"**. The next level of adaptability is in push-hands where you learn to blend with your partner and adapt to their push and pull as it were…. I use the term **'constant contact'** rather than blend as it feels better to me but that's just words, ultimately what you are looking for (or sensing for) is your partners lack of adaptability to the interplay of push-hands and in turn your adaptability to respond to the opportunity. Hey, if in doubt you could try the banana trade.

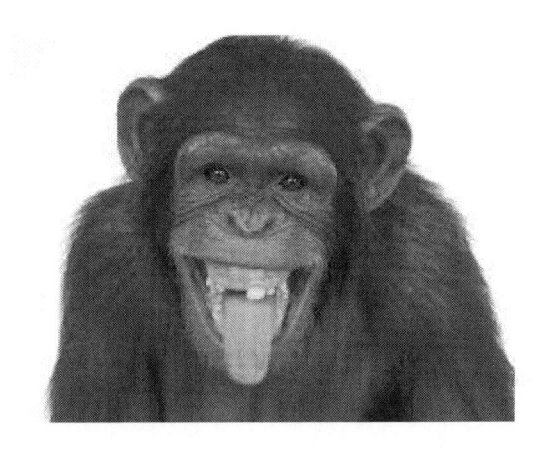

I wonna banana..!!

Pearls Of Wisdom Advice From My Mother !

My mom passed away age 97 years. She was not an intellectual in the strict sense of the word, but I think she gave me advice to get through life in a much easier to use scenario than it would have been if she was.
Although nothing to do with Tai Chi I thought I would share them with you as the newsletter can always use good common sense and humour.———

1. The world values you at your OWN valuation. (always be confident of your ability to succeed in whatever you want in life, and let others see it.)
2. If money becomes the most important think in your life you will never be truly happy (or rich)
3. Never envy anyone anything.
4. Never tell lies, especially if you haven't a good memory!
5. Always help older people (she encouraged me to carry elderly neighbours shopping home for them from a really young age,) and this empathy with the older person has stayed with me.
6. You need to keep mobile, it keeps you alive and healthy.
7. Never spoil a child, no one likes spoilt children.
8. If you cannot afford to pay cash for something, Don't have it! Save up, then get it.
9. If a man ever goes to hit you, hit him FIRST!
10. Don't examine relationships too closely, you will just get more confused! (advise she gave my daughter when she asked her for advice and opinion on a new boyfriend)

And to finish, 2 more gems I love—
After watching a James Bond film in her 90s she turned to me and said *"I think he is a bit promiscuous, don't you!"*
"Don't wash your hair when you have your period, it will send you mad!" Obviously I did not take heed to that one
Please share with us advice from your mom.... I look forward to reading and sharing it.

The History Of Boading Balls

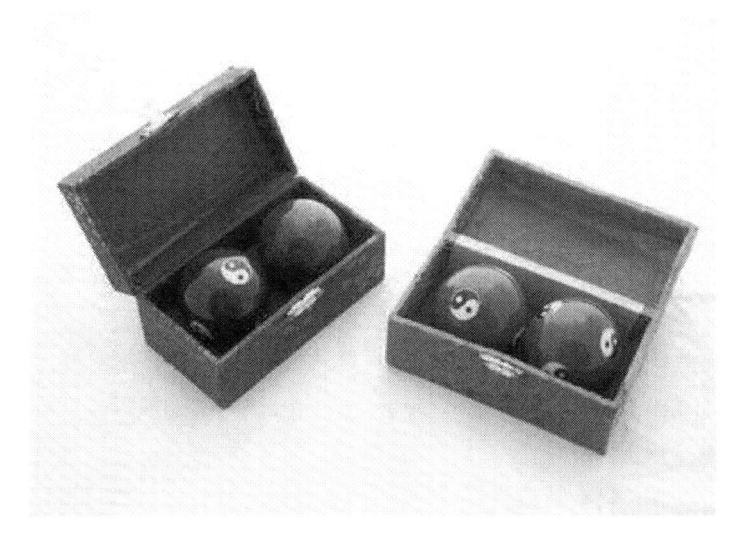

We have all seen those nicely presented boxes containing a duo of small metal balls painted or enamelled with attractive designs, very often the Yin and Yang symbols or Dragons etc and many give off a very pleasant "chime" as you roll them around in the palm of your hand.
But do you know they are called Boading balls or the history of their origin? If you don't then read on for enlightenment.
Today they are more still popular, riding the wave of Feng Shui popularity.
Boading balls are said to be one of the 3 treasures of Boading City (no one ever says what the other two are).
Known as the South Gate of Beijing, it lies smack in the centre of a golden triangle formed by huge metropolises of Beijing, Tianjin and Shijiazhuang.
Although iron balls go back to the Song Dynasty (960-1127 CE), according to legend, it was a Boading blacksmith in the Ming Dynasty (1368-1644 CE) that first created the chime-filled balls as instructed by the gods in a dream.
Thus Boading laid claim to all balls, chime filled or not.

The Emperor was so impressed that he commissioned these balls exclusively for the imperial family. It was much later when they fell into the hands of us commoners!
Now you can't find a Chinatown shop that lacks these balls anywhere.
Using Boading balls is very simple.
Just spin the balls in your palm. If you really want to show your skill, don't let the balls touch!!!.Or you can just rub the balls together constantly.
If you become skilled with 2 balls it is suggested you advance to spinning up to 5 balls at a time.
There is even a unique form of contact juggling today using these balls, most notably demonstrated by artist Michael Moschen in the 1986 film LABYRINTH starring David Bowie and Jennifer Connelly.

According to traditional Chinese medicine, spinning Boading balls stimulates many significant acupressure points within the hand, helping relieve all sorts of maladies believed to be due to "improper qi" flow.

Today this has been translated into a panacea for everything from high blood pressure, carpel tunnel syndrome, warding off the common cold! And the soothing chime is marketed in this age of stress as an anxiety reliever.

As a testament to its health giving virtues, the average lifespan of a Boading citizen is 6.4 years longer than the rest of China.
The balls can come in many forms, solid metal, cloisonné, crystal and some even made from jade and other semi-precious stones.
And this is a case where size matters!!! Small ones are for multiple ball spinning while big ones are for big fat hands.
As they come in pairs they were also sometimes given as a lucky wedding gift.
So why it is also regarded as a weapon?

Chinese used to carry Boading balls all the time.

Imagine being hit in the face. This alone was enough to justify their inclusion in the classical Chinese lists of throwing weapons.

So now you know the facts surrounding these balls maybe the next time you see them you might be tempted to buy a pair to sit and spin whilst watching the telly eating a slice of chocolate cake but justifying it by spinning your balls to improve your health!!! And if anyone says otherwise stick to your story!

Here is a little story to amuse –

"In 1972, the Chinese presented President Nixon (they did it to Regan too) with Boading balls as a quaint "cultural exchange" gift. It was a simple ploy.

Give the "gift" then sit back and watch as he struggled to maintain presidential dignity, fumbling with his balls at the dinner table. Of course, any Chinese dignitary can whip his balls about like there's no tomorrow Ball spinning is a common skill amongst Chinese.

Nothing like iron balls to cool down cold war diplomacy"

Printed in Great Britain
by Amazon